M000189041

Living in My Afterlife

Living in My Afterlife

An invisible disability and health odyssey affecting millions

Robert Feuerstein

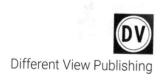

Different View Publishing

Copyright © 2021 by Robert Feuerstein

All rights reserved. No part of this book may be reproduced in any form by mechanical or electronic means, including information storage and retrieval systems, without permission in writing from the publisher, except by a reviewer or researcher who may quote brief passages in a review or scholarly publication with author credits. Every effort to comply with copyright requirements has been made by seeking permission and acknowledging owners of source material used in the text.

Disclaimer:
i) This book is a collection of memories. The personal stories and memories by individuals recorded here are their version of events and have been both provided and reproduced in good faith with no disrespect or defamation intended. Every effort has been made to ensure the researched information is correct. No liability for incorrect information or factual errors will be accepted by the author.
ii) The views and opinions expressed in this work are solely those of the author. Some names may have been changed to protect privacy; however, they reflect real people and events.

Cover and interior layout: Pickawoowoo Publishing Group
Cover illustration: Canstockphoto by ZdenekSasek

Different View Publishing
Library of Congress Control Number: 2021918270
First Printing, 2021
ISBN: 978-1-7378847-0-5 (paperback)
ISBN: 978-1-7378847-1-2 (ebook)

TO THE 70 MILLION DYSAUTONOMIA SUFFERERS.
COURAGEOUS VICTIMS OF AN INVISIBLE,
MISUNDERSTOOD, DISEASE:

I SEE YOU.

"...Who can stop the rain?
Who can stop the rain from falling?
Who can stop this pain that's drowning me?"

Thompson Twins

CONTENTS

CONTENTS

I have a dilemma that far too many people will experience, if they haven't already. My age-old predicament is older than Hamlet's "To be or not to be" Alive? Do I want to continue living the rest of my life in my condition? Do I even have the freedom to determine how I live the end of my life? And what kind of counterproductive and conflicting health system did we get trapped in? But don't dare tell those who maintain this unsustainable system.

1

FAIR WARNING

My misery began with an innocuous cough.

Like most of us who get a bad winter's cold, I tried to endure, believing, "sure, this'll pass." But like the frog in a pot of water slowly coming to a boil, I had no idea what was happening.

In retrospect, I came to realize this was also the beginning of an ordeal that would transform me from a healthy 69-year-old ex-home builder, following a late-in-life passion as a restaurant owner, into a spastic individual playing bumper cars off of walls with my body.

Six months later, I could hardly get out of bed and my skin had turned yellow in appearance. I didn't have an appetite; my body was tingly all over, and, as I discovered, I was afflicted with an illness that has the medical community completely baffled. A case that would stump even *House, M.D.*

Yet, I'm not alone in my quandary. Similar stories happen every year to an unimaginable number of people who randomly get snared in the best medical system on Earth—or so we're led to believe. Currently there are millions of sufferers, the world over, experiencing one derivative or another of this illness. And all they seem to be able to do is just get by. But, "lucky" me, I've also got something extra special.

I feel like I'm stuck looking up my own butt, immobile in life, and wondering if there's another way out. Not a good place to be.

But after a debilitating, acute illness, I thought: "What were my choices to solve this dilemma?" How would I navigate my future in this condition?

Before the onset of this affliction, I was a happy guy. I wouldn't exchange my life for another. So, with this abrupt change in events, I started thinking about my choices. No way was I going to continue living like this. It's Hamlet's, "Do I, or Don't I?" It's a dilemma of the human condition and nature's perfectly created system that there will be no escapees. But, while we seek the extension of human life, we inadvertently create numerous conundrums contrary to that system.

So then, how does one, in my position, sit down with their family to discuss ending their life? How does someone, when they look perfectly normal and healthy, and they believe there's no way to continue, or relief from their new situation, even explain the conditions they have to endure in order to continue on living for the complacency of others.

If I can pave the way to open up such an emotional, end-of-life conversation, sooner than later, about the inevitable ALL of us will confront; to me, that's worth the time to discuss it. But don't be fooled by my appearance, I'm just a regular guy suffering a universal human dilemma.

* * *

About 18 months ago I was Robert version 3.0. Someone who always felt ageless despite being, chronologically, 69. Today I feel like an over eighty-year-old, down-graded, less-sophisticated, boring model. What pile of shit did I step in that my new life comes down to this? The transformed me is not pretty. And yet, the surrealistic thing is that looking at me hardly any physical change is noticeable. People say I look wonderful. But what's going on under the skin is something out of the *Twilight Zone*. The only tell-tale giveaway is what's immediately revealed from my side: a medically induced, marsupial bulge. Yet, I have a closet full of unwearable, skinny-man clothes, with, of all now-dreaded things, zippers and buttons!

* * *

My radical transformation kept me in a hospital for three months. When I was finally released, there was no definitive diagnosis or prognosis for recovery. Number 500, or so they said, at The Mayo Clinic in Minnesota. An LGi1 autoimmune, induced neuropathy (whatever *that* means), that no one can explain. Although I have my suspicions.

For those not familiar with neuropathy, think about when your hand, foot, leg, or arm "falls asleep," your limb feels rubbery and numb with the pins and needles feeling. It'll take a while, but as blood recirculates to the affected area, the prickliness and deadness go away. Then, back to "business as usual."

Mine started one day and progressed from my feet to my neck. The Myelin sheath on my nerves were literally fried and now I'm a caged, tortured prisoner in my own body. And oh, did I mention, when this all began, I was two days away from a liver transplant?

* * *

Every Monday, Wednesday, and Friday, now some 200 days into this ordeal, I roll out a colored, putty, playdough-type material, place pennies on the dough, and press them in, only to then dig them out again with my fingers, and again, and again... This, supposedly, to regain my strength and dexterity. No, I'm not drooling, and it won't come down to that if I have anything to do with it.

As a builder, author, restaurateur, dad to three boys, and a husband, of course I had nothing better to do or places to be in the latter part of my life. This is what retirement has come down to? If you ask me, this putty 'n pennies business is not making me any stronger or yielding any encouragement to continue to exist. So, if this is my life going forward, I have many things to think about. Some not so pleasant, even taboo by some standards.

* * *

Before June of 2018, I was a healthy, 69-year-old, occasional Cialis user suffering a persistent cough. I was just like that middle-aged guy who left his "Wall St."-type job to have a farm raising goats. Or sort of...My farm was a restaurant. Just different goats. I wanted to cook the type of food that my friends raved and goaded me on about when we entertained.

So, big-shot me, I opened a restaurant.

It didn't take much convincing. After spending about 40 years in the building and development business of housing, I saw the hand-writing on the wall. Those days were coming to an end. Although building was my first love, I was getting tired of the routine: the early hours, the continuous challenges of the economy's ups and downs, finicky homeowners, the younger subcontractors and their new "games." Every day it was a new "Excedrin headache."

I remembered my days as a kid smoking ribs, ducks, and chickens. Flying out the back door of the house with a pot of water to squelch a fire in our old brick fireplace smoker in the backyard was part of the routine. Fire was the enemy, smoke the pleasure. That's what creates the low-temperature cooking method I loved. So, some fifty years later, I wanted to lay down the construction plans and return to the roots of my ambition and memories.

Spontaneously, my dreams would go up in "Smoked." I built my restaurant around a focus on a different kind of BBQ. Fewer tables, healthier food with my low-salt and low-sugar recipes, and specializing more for take-out and catering; the wife and I loved the different foods from traveling and entertaining.

The opening and operation of this restaurant would be challenging for a novice. But I wasn't afraid. My naiveté always spared me from anxiety. I was simply responding to my complimentary guest's encouragement. So, from the design and construction, to organizing menus, recipes, and staff, procuring materials, food supplies, and equipment, it was all familiar. On top of that, I would also find myself doing the food shopping, prep, and cooking for hours in the kitchen. The pencils and paper, the calculations; although I was in heaven, I, also, found myself washing the pots 'n pans in a three-compartment sink too many times when the help didn't show. I discovered running a restaurant, at my age, was maybe a little too ambitious, but determined, nevertheless, to overcome the issues in the pursuit of success. Unfortunately, I would also learn and experience what most have realized in their lifetimes—"shit happens."

* * *

By June of 2018, I was a candidate for a liver transplant in one of NYC's major transplant hospitals. That's when my life and the lives of everyone around me abruptly changed.

Just stop what you're doing and go to room 701 in the hospital. The door to that room, for me, turned out to be a portal to another life, and I was to accept the changed "itinerary" for the rest of my existence. Not just for me, but my family too. No one had a choice or say in the matter, and, basically, I just dumped it all on them. I don't wish any of this on anyone. What would all of this mean? What were to be the implications for the cast of characters involved in my life?

My illness presents symptoms of unknown origin and complexity. This is the central issue that drives the machinations of the medical system that would dominate my life from then on while I managed the family, running an ongoing business, and dwindling funds. Diagnosis, treatment, patient's care and rights came to occupy my mind. A spaghetti-bowl of issues, for sure.

How did I manage to survive 12 weeks in the hospital? Each day was 24 hours long starting at around 4am. Every day it was something else, which, all taken together, led me to believe something of an unknown, earthquake-sized event in my life could be unfolding. Perhaps I even stepped into a deeper pile of mystery dung than most. The final scene in the movie, *Deliverance*, is where the valley is flooded, and a hand breaks the surface of the water. You know there's a bigger narrative attached that's below the surface. So, permit me to get to my story. I've got more to tell than what's on display. And it's "Do I, or Don't I?"

2

The story

It was back in December of 2017 when the dominos of my life-changing events began to fall. It was as simple as that cough that wouldn't quit, despite pristine nonsmoker's lungs. It could be quite violent at times, even causing convulsions and loss of breath. And I just had a flu shot. I speculated it was from the shot: "Maybe I should go to the doctor?" I told myself, playing self-doctor. It's been five years since seeing one. I'll just get a Z-Pack (Azithromycin: an antibacterial medication.) and clear it up like in the past, right?

No such luck.

Now, more than a year and a half later, I'm beholden to others doing some tasks for me. I'm not in control of certain events, relegating me to waiting for others. I find most people are considerate. I can tell because my "thank you" meter is spinning all of the time.

Thanks for holding the door.

Thanks for getting wheelchairs.

Thanks for helping to put on jackets.

Thanks for this, for that, for everything!

Maybe I should just get a sign and hang it around my neck.

I give them the tacit nod-wave, as they hold the door, or wait in their cars at the crosswalks, observing me hobble across the street, while I imagine them muttering: "Better he than I." Not my usual

M.O. I feel like my body has become that of an old man when my brain says otherwise. Now, I'm a doee, not a doer.

Being 70 was only a number to me. Last year I was a "bounce-around." Now, I practically crawl on a cane or walker. But I also represent a population of the newly undefined or elderly who become stricken with similar issues all too frequently, and all too randomly. The easy shit is fixable. But what about the stuff that can't be explained, or easily treated?

I will not be a Head-in-the-Bed because nobody has a clue, I will not.

With whatever illness I was brewing, I imagined myself ending up as that poor soul suffering from Locked-in Syndrome after a stroke in *The Diving Bell and the Butterfly,* wherein the victim was confined to a bed, paralyzed, except for the ability to blink one eye, and even able to author a book. The constant undercurrent in my hospital bed is that if my illness progresses or the prognosis is poor, I can't see how I continue to be a burden on everyone.

Hospital stays aren't cheap. Observation, medication, tests, and treatment all amount to staggering bills in the American Healthcare System. My illness is an invisible jail-cell of an affliction. How much do I have to pay to continue on living to endure for the pleasure of others in such a cell? A woman said she wouldn't want me to end my life because she wanted to enjoy my humor, wisdom, and knowledge. I said, "I'm not here for your pleasure AND at my expense!"

They make you have babies against your will, make you pay for healthcare, tell you to go to war, and then with all this misery and possibly more, you're told to endure it for the rest of your natural life. Only eleven states currently permit an 'end of life' option and that's only if you're going to die within 6 months. Isn't it a cruel and unusual punishment to keep one alive under such ongoing duress; and maybe just because of the luck of the draw with qualified doctors?! We treat our pets with more consideration. We, at least, euthanize them!

Fortunately, I feel my life is full enough of satisfaction and accomplishment. I'm thrilled with my children, my wife, and the life we lived. No secret girlfriends to mourn my passing. In short, my life is a long and well lived one. Maybe even boring to some. How much more could I do that I would lament not doing, dead OR alive?

My bucket list was self-designed, not by some magazine or movie star. I could be content with the simple pleasure of walking around a farmer's market, smelling and touching the fresh produce. The fragrance of a ripe peach was intoxicating to me. I built my houses, wrote a book and built a restaurant and catering business. A friend commented that: "I appeared to be comfortable in my own skin." I put smiles of satisfaction on once-stranger's faces. I could read the critical reviews or pass by my work, reminisce, and say, with my heart glowing: "See, I did that." Not like some garment designer whose latest creation has long been thrown in the trash or a stockbroker's last trade; there and gone.

My wife, Dee, and I traveled, ate well enough, and enjoyed each other along with our ups and downs. Hey, who doesn't? But the game has changed. I'm handicapped with a bizarre illness—and I have the car sticker to confirm it! I've done my hard work. Now, time to enjoy. Only, I'm in no position to enjoy as much, if at all.

Now, this is a less than zero-sum game. I don't believe I have much more to contribute or accomplish. I know a family is all about love, but I feel like I've become a net drain on my family. Long gone are the days of my feeling in-charge.

Hard working, American success story ends as a Head-in-the-Bed. Body unwilling and unable to continue to force even a TV remote control to follow commands. The family and employees contain their pity. The only difference is that this story also harbors both anger and fear.

What is one of the things one does when confronting an acute precipitous decline like mine? An article caught my attention in *The NY Times*: "A debate over rational suicide."

I'm a practical guy. What's ahead for me?

Some would say I'm angry or depressed to even consider terminating my life. But this thought is as logical as any I have ever considered. What is logical about being driven crazy out of one's mind and continue existing in this torture cage? Or worse yet, as my neuropathy progresses unabated, what worse condition might I find myself in, someday, than I am now?

Overall, it's just looking at the cost vs. reward. It doesn't seem to add up to hang around waiting for cookies with unborn grandkids. If I got hit by a car and my life was over quickly, the wife would have the life insurance in the bank, the "sympathy" cards would be in a box in the closet, and the lox 'n bagels would be long cleaned up. All would be moving on.

Instead, she has a flat-footed, needy, hobbled individual in her midst. More of a burden than before, and the uncrowned, new title of "Caregiver." All I can think is: "Now, how much ya love me?" Our deck of cards has been reshuffled.

Like the downhill skier, Lindsey Vaughn says, "It's time to listen to my body—and it's the time to say goodbye." Sure, she's only talking about retiring from a sport. I'm talking about retiring my need for most everything except a good, hot, crematorium.

But before you pass judgement on me, let me explain what I'm afflicted with.

I have just about full-body neuropathy from my toes to my neck and shoulders. That includes peripheral neuropathy, including arms and legs, truncal neuropathy, which extends from the waist to the shoulders. The truncal part of this illness is rare and feels like I'm wearing a bulletproof vest tight to the body, 24/7. Even walking is now a challenge. This is in addition to the autonomic affects, the body's involuntary movements, which include: urination difficulty, digestion and gastrointestinal issues, low blood-pressure leading to fainting, decreased smell and consequential lack of taste, poor balance and loss of strength in legs, sex drive, and the inability to achieve an erection; and more.

You. Have. No. Idea.

My body is going in different directions, all the time.

A sex life? Fuhgeddaboudit. No dose of Cialis could wake up that drooping puppy, not to mention the, sometimes, gymnastics required.

But little of my body, now, works as it did for 69 years. What do I have to look forward to, but a seat in a circus sideshow? "Come see the Head-in-the-Bed."

Last but not least, my "executive function" is also affected. My thought process suffers because planning, working memory (RAM), time management, and organization is slowed down.

How does one have a discussion or an argument when they can't even remember the previous thought?! I feel like I have to learn to paint with my toes. Just another level of difficulty to overcome. Because I'm not only able to write with a little more than blinking an eye, like the *Diving Bell* guy...Should I feel luckier, nevertheless?

Everyone assures me that my condition is not life threatening. But ending my life might be better. I ask: "Is being confined in chains acceptable to slaves, to prisoners, to the tortured?" Enslaved parents were known to kill their children rather than they live under the oppression of slavery. Was this my punishment for taking a bowling ball home from the alley, on my bike, at age ten? Even though, in the 1950's, it was "fashionable" to steal monogrammed cloth napkins from the "friendly skies" of the airlines; a spoon here and there from your local restaurant; soap and engraved towels from fancy hotels; and plenty of other souvenirs of a trip? I only heisted a bowling ball! They didn't have #PilferinLife or #AcceptablePilfering" back then!

Yet, I'm a science-based guy; no unfounded hopes or prayers here. I don't think I've ever been accused of being some chicken without a head and that's exactly what I would be, desperately, running around seeking some magic elixir that probably doesn't even exist. Therefore, in my case, where's the trust or reasoned optimism for recovery; the reason to continue living?

And then, of course, when the news is shared with others, everyone's got a cure. Friends, relatives, and even strangers all chime in with miracle cures; some exotic, to others, some more mundane. Among them: Acupuncture, vitamins, massages, chiropractic, pot, and CBD oils; maybe even electro-therapy of some sort; and countless numbers of self-help, cures. One very seriously suggested, "Hey, have you tried a hyperbaric chamber?" Except there's only one problem. There's basically no science for any cures, except, so I've faintly heard, some possible slight, nerve regeneration on its own. But so far, all to no avail. It's all gossip.

What keeps me alive suffering in this condition when there may only be fluke stories of recovery? Facebook friends groups are loaded with moms frantically searching for their kid's treatments, and the elderly wandering through a jungle of almost useless remedies. But it's just not my style to travel through life with a blindfold on and hang out for mere "hope."

To me, hope is as productive as sitting on a bench in a snowstorm, at midnight, waiting for a bus, *after* a State of Emergency has been declared. To me, there're fewer situations of being alone.

There's a price to pay with this affliction. Of course, I want to see certain projects through, especially with my three sons on their way into adulthood, but it's costly to have faith in a blind alley for eight months or two years plus, waiting for some, maybe, "miracle cure" for nerve regeneration, that may never come!

Sure, I could spend umpteen dollars in search of some unproven remedy promoted by some unverifiable monk hiding in the Himalayas using Amazon shipping, but most probably it would also be out-of-pocket, for Medicare wouldn't reimburse a fantasy chase. What's my longevity with this illness? What's my life-expectancy at this point? I could use all my remaining life waiting, hoping, hanging around for relief, a cure—and then still die of some other natural causes! F'k that!

Am I, or for that matter, most others, so important that the state will pay carte blanchě to any doc with a bill? The answer for me is no. The end of all our lives are going to happen sooner or later and the world will get along. For me, how many, profoundly, memorable statements can come out of my mouth that I should live another day? And who should bear the cost?

The cause of my affliction is idiopathic—or, in other words, unknown. But just because the cause of something isn't known doesn't mean that there is no cause. It's just unknown or unacceptable because currently it doesn't make sense to the medical community. The same as the earth was, once, considered the center of the universe—until, for more convincing reasons, it wasn't. (In spite of those like the Flat Earthers.)

But there was a confluence of events in my case that is too coincidental to ignore. So, the timeline of my story begins with that slow, unsuspecting crawl, to the top of a roller coaster-ride to come. And who knows who that unsuspecting next rider could be. Are you feeling invincible, perhaps?

* * *

In pursuit of treating that cough that started in December 2017, I went to my internist requesting a Z-Pack. That's a 5-day antibiotic used to knock out infections. It didn't work, and about two months later, after returning from a trip, worn out, I returned to him. He prescribed Augmentin this time. Just my luck, THAT didn't work either.

He couldn't help, so this appeared to be the job of a pulmonologist. The cough was horrendous—so much so that I could just about pass out from the convulsions. The lung gunk was winning.

The new doctor gave me a battery of tests. Breathing in and out was torture. I wasn't in any capacity to play around with those breath measuring devices while coughing up a fit. You're told to blow, blow, blow, and blow into this tube until your eyeballs pop out of your head. Richard Simmons couldn't cheer-lead any better.

When the doctor reviewed the results, he said it was a nasty virus, and prescribed steroids, inhalers, and took me off the Augmentin. "Sounds like a plan," I said.

A couple of weeks later there was improvement in my chest and cough, so Doc weaned me off the steroids. That was like April, but my "friend," the cough, returned shortly thereafter. Was it too early to decrease the steroids?

Pulmonologist said, "Return to an internist." Maybe I had allergies. One white flag raised on this battlefield.

Mick Jagger's "I can't get no satisfaction" swirls in my head.

A new internist prescribed Augmentin—again—and said, "Return in a couple of weeks." My new equivalent of: "Take two and call me in the morning." Wouldn't you know, no improvements. Now, to get really tough, he then doubled down on the dosage. Dork head.

I wanted relief and I was going to my youngest son, Landon's, college graduation in Vermont that coming weekend. How dare *I* question the Doctor? Trusting sheep usually don't doubt their doctor. Right?

I should have. Apparently, *my* doctor wasn't aware of some bulletin in the medical community—which I would learn later on while Googling—about possible adverse reactions to increased or continued dosage of this common antibiotic. That would become a telltale marker in my case. Who sends up the red flag for these bulletins and how is it disseminated? Not to mention does anybody adhere to the recommendations.

So, maybe there was some connection to the repeated use of the antibiotic Augmentin and my condition. No one's sure. No hands raised accepting responsibility. Nevertheless, it became a piece in my soon-to-be puzzle.

That, as it turns out, became that high point when the "ride" was going to start.

It could happen to anyone. Why would you think you're invincible? Sinclair Lewis', Frank Zappa, and others: "It can't happen here?" Until it does!

3

Graduation

I felt horrible that weekend—dragging my ass all over Vermont. I didn't want to ruin anybody's party, but I'm sure I may have been doing a pretty good job of it anyway. I didn't want to get out of my hotel bed, dragging my ass to all the celebratory activities. And I really didn't want to tell anyone, of my ailment, for fear of raining on the "parade." But the last straw was that I couldn't eat—one of my favorite activities, even though I could have been distracted by a beautiful restaurant on the water!

So, we drove home quietly. I was celebrating the last of the long car trips, the end of the tuition and living expense payments! A big graduation, hurray for Landon!! A muted hurray for us!!

Landon would be staying behind in Vermont a few more days to say his goodbyes before returning home—to live with Mom and Dad. No hurray for him. But not long after, he would have a home-party for friends and family, and then be off to Israel for a graduation break before returning home and looking for a job.

But something still didn't feel right with me. I felt the double dose of the antibiotic wasn't working—so I decided to not continue taking it. And one day later, after we took Landon to the airport, I felt it was time to go to an emergency room. This eagle had crash-landed.

* * *

I sensed that all the doctors for the last six months were not getting me anywhere. Schlepping my ass around, loss of appetite, wanting to crawl up and sleep forever, and from what I would be told later, turning yellow, just didn't seem quite the normal behavior for what I was used to experiencing, for "a healthy guy" who had experienced little more, in his life, than a prophylactic pill for high cholesterol and a routine hernia operation. So, I reported my symptoms to the emergency room attendant, and at the end of the examination and report, I was told: "There's nothing wrong enough with you to keep you overnight." and that I would be discharged to go home, tingling and all in the body. Waaaaat?

Nothing wrong? WTF? Most of us know that feeling when we're getting the run-around from a wrong answer. The wife practically begged for me to stay and be observed. I was ready to point a scalpel at my temple and pull the trigger. Finally, we reached my, then, current internist (Doctor double-down), who arranged to admit me. Maybe *he* felt a ping of pain. Apparently, being a squeaky wheel in this case got some results. Well, after two days of more tests in the hospital, and after some young residents concluded I was a patient in over my head at this facility, I was being transported, and on my way, to one of the top hospitals in NYC as a candidate for a liver transplant!! The coaster was now on *its* way too—careening downhill!!!! My "iceberg" lay straight ahead.

Imagine, two days before, maybe soon to be dead, (and maybe a missed opportunity) I was inadmissible to a hospital in my condition.

What ensued from then on, would all be alien to me. Transported to some only heard-about hospital, liver failure? Whatever was coming would be a first for me, but whatever, it just wasn't registering in my brain. Wasn't I invincible, "The clock that keeps on ticking?" The bunny rabbit that wouldn't quit, relatively ageless? "Young at heart?" Doesn't this only happen to other people that you read or hear about? Helloooo, wake-up callllll. "Hey, did you hear that "Boomer" Feuerstein's got this crazy-ass illness? Honey, let's take the family for a walk in the woods." Not anymore for me. My new destination was coming into focus.

It was a warm, late-Spring, early evening and I was all alone watching the landmarks fly by from the back of the transport van. All too familiar landmarks to occupy and ease a nervous mind and help determine my route to the city. "Why were they going this way when there were shorter routes?" as they flew by with my peering out of the little window of the rear door. But it didn't matter. I would still end up at the place they had destined for me. A place that would investigate my human beingness from an anatomical perspective starting from my toes to my scalp, inside and out. All necessary to figure out what was ailing me.

So, they took me out of the ambulance and those wheels popped down to maintain the stretcher at an elevated height. You know the type you see other people on in the news, and in we went, into my strange and unfamiliar home for the next three months.

It certainly wasn't the decor I was used to.

But did I know what was in store for me? Hardly! And I felt alone, while watching it all from a distance. I just couldn't relate any more than the wonderment of a six-year-old experiences going to the zoo and seeing all the animals. This was like a fourth-grade field trip.

WTF was I doing in this place for *sick* people? It's a place I thought only grandparents frequented.

After arriving at the NYC hospital, my first room would be on the 7th floor for observation. Relieved that I would finally be getting some serious attention, the thought of a liver transplant, although scary, was certainly not mentally clicking as to the implications. They're going to cut my belly open, big scar? Is this going to be one of those jokes that I'll crave different food, or speak a different language depending on who the donor is? But to make it perfectly clear for a perfectly "healthy" guy with little hospital experience, how would I know what to expect? And all without a "welcome" cocktail—mini-parasol and all?! Imagine!

On that beautiful, warm, late-spring evening, patient admitted, to a humongous, multi-entranced, 12-story, innocuous-people buzzing around, major health facility; *"presenting"* (as they say) with liver failure, cirrhosis among other things, along with tingling sensation throughout the body, (and a possibly undeveloped and immature brain, too. Ha!), and a candidate for a liver transplant, for sure, my bilirubin was about 10—when normal was less than 1. That was early evening. This was me.

My first introduction to a hospital-stay came the next morning—at the second dream-hour of 4:30 am. Blood giving time! One vial for you, two vials for them, and another bunch for all the rest of the others. My precious blood was being given away. "Now, go back to sleep." said this middle-of-the-night, blood-sucking creature. "Okay, I'll try to go back to sleep." But I rustled for another two hours; "What was I doing here, and what will come next?"

Nope! At 7a.m., with a shift change, the nursing staff would introduce themselves as was the practice every day for all patients—evvvvry day. That wasn't amusing for long. They now do 12-hour shifts, three times a week for expediency. They love to erase the earlier shift's name from the chalkboard and write their own—as if they were something special, some with a personal touch, and certainly with a smile. But who cares? Sick people who think they're on their deathbed, with a "fried" liver to-go without onions, are not interested in smiley faced nurses. *You* can't smile enough to make *me* feel better!

Only, now, oops, 7:30a.m., time for breakfast. 8a.m.—time for the first explorers to visit—those wannabe student-doctors instructed to ask plenty of questions, all to be shared with the attendings of each discipline in pursuit of the ever-elusive diagnosis. Now, realizing I'm in room 701 overlooking some atrium courtyard and visited by a battery of doctors, I say, casually, thinking I'd like to get off of this "zoo trip" and back to work: "What's up doc? What's wrong with me?" That answer would be as elusive as chasing a feather in the wind.

The army of doctors: The liver team, heart, kidneys, blood, and on and on, each with its own exotic and official sounding title, some with jumbled letters, that aren't even in the alphabet, in their titles, imagined just to confuse the patient. All to set out on their scavenger hunt, on a pertinent facts find, to offer opinions on what was this patient's problem. I felt like I was a patient in the book: "*Spots on the Wall*: by Who Flung Poo." Yay or nay on cancer, heart issue, blood problem, or any other possible diagnosis hidden in the medical annals of illnesses—just to see what stuck. They all huddled and conferred: Dr. Yo, Dr. ko, Dr. McGuire, Dr. Brown, Dr. Yellow, Dr. Purple, Dr. Ali, Dr. Vizolli, Dr. Toy, Dr. Male, Dr. female, and all the others lurking in between, along with an endless representation of, paint-bucket-swirled-looking, potpourri of international doctors all wanting to take a whack at uncoiling my spaghetti-bowl of an illness. And THAT, at first blush, which would appear, as an understatement, and confusing, would be awhile. But I don't want to be someone's Guinea-pig patient so they can learn. Or do I? Do I even have a say in the matter?

The students swarmed with the residents using me as the study-ragdoll-of-the-day. A perplexing presentation of liver failure and soon-to-be-realized, neuropathy. "Does this hurt?" "Follow my finger." As if I were in a bubble, "press your arms outward, up, sideways," as they pushed parts of my body, testing for strength. The list of tests from blood to cat scans, MRI's, EKG's, EEG's and an alphabet soup of more tests, poking, blood-drawing, etc. was unleashed to search for an explanation of my condition. Little did they all realize this was the early stages of my ordeal. Is *any* shit sticking?

They even put me on a nebulizer, an inhalation device administering medication to the lungs, thinking it would help. How, in retrospect, so pedestrian and feeble. Like using a Q-Tip to mop the floor. Hematologists, pulmonologists, infectious disease specialists, neurologists and every other medical discipline chimed in with the wadabouts, suggestions, and prescribed tests to either confirm or deny a suspected diagnosis only to be discarded. I felt a gaggle of washwomen made more sense. Where *is* "*House*" when you need him?" Overwhelming is an understatement. "Humpty Dumpty fell on the floor...," I thought, but all were having trouble figuring out how to put Humpty, Bob back together again!

So, the tests continued, more cat scans, MRI's, blood tests every morning starting at 4am—and more just to make sure. There's no rest in a hospital. Testing for cancer, to pneumonia, to GB, MG, MS, the immediate tell-all defied classification because some component of the diagnosis was missing; all while further compounded with an unknown overlay of a liver issue. They take vitals every four hours if not more. They wake you to take blood-pressure, blood samples, feed you breakfast, lunch and dinner—if they get the order right, tests, residents, interns, nurses, meal-order people, maintenance staff—an endless entourage of hospital personnel enough to man an aircraft carrier. They don't care if they wake or disturb you. That concern is not in their "playbook." They've got their jobs to attend to. **A hospital is not a place for rest.** It's a place where their business is to do their own jobs, and maybe by the way, treat or heal "frog"-people like us! After you— "next frog. Er, patient."

In the first hospital, two glasses wine a day was originally proffered as a cause of my liver failure. I was, consequently, "labeled," an alcoholic, after reminding myself of some elementary school story, the *Scarlet Letter*. But Dr. Toy offered in the "big-city" hospital, the perfect retort— "Who's *not* having two glasses a day? Otherwise, we're *all* alcoholics!" Reassuring light moments to save the day from some over-eager beaver wannabee residents.

Meanwhile, back with me in my room the second day in, now I'm trying to make sense of it all as to hospital procedure, and realizing I'm tethered to an IV pole that will follow me around—like to the bathroom. So off we'll go, my pole with the IV bottle and I, (ha, ha!) only to realize that I'm in the hospital for some apparent, unknown, and significant reason. As I get out of bed and I'm holding my pole (now, not funny), the room quickly gets dizzy and down I go. Crash on the floor. Now I'm a hospital statistic— "Help, I've fallen." Something I can't remember *ever* doing. But now certainly a member of the hospital's watch list—a "fall candidate"—apparently what will figure out on that front would be a hospital's *Achilles Heel*.

By all means, CYA (cover your ass) and make sure a patient doesn't fall. Even if staff is turned into paranoid practitioners. So, with that news, after the start of the battery of tests, and a couple of days later, I was transferred to a private room, number 906 East, overlooking the *Hell Gate* and *RFK bridges*. Hmmm, not bad for a Medicare patient. It's a private room with a dramatic view. I couldn't be happier. But also, not realizing, these rooms were like, and as expensive as "hen's teeth." This is Mt. Saini, a major, renowned, New York City health facility. But actually, I was being isolated because they didn't know if I was either infected or infectious. Maybe not such great news.

As the staff were now all wearing masks, I was told I was either potentially toxic, or others were toxic to me—but that couldn't be determined, yet. So, the private room dream, and the battery of tests lasted about a week until a real paying patient showed up and, after concluding no one's catching even a cold from me, I was booted to another room—this time an outside bed and with a roommate. In a semi-private room with two beds, when the curtains are drawn for privacy, the bed closest to the window is the outside bed and the other bed, closest to the bathroom, could be a closet in Nairobi.

Another first: I would realize that this roommate patient was a moaner. But hey, wait, how did I get to be in a room with someone who makes so much noise that they would keep me awake at night? Who *makes* so much noise? And, in this whole hospital, who was sicker than I? On top of that, what did I know about a personal experience with death other than my father dying some 30 years earlier and my mom recently of the ripe old, withering, age of 94?

Not to be rude or unsympathetic, but I didn't think this was the time for chivalry. Or maybe nobody cared. But I selfishly had my own problems brewing. Now, it was *Curb Your Enthusiasm*-style, mano-a-mano in my book. Who could make the other quiet? He certainly didn't respond to my requests. So, I was going to "over-loud" my TV over the moaning of this roommate into submission.

Well, I certainly won that contest. They wheeled him out the next day, with a sheet over his head. How did I know he was on the way out—literally?! Did I have something to do with his demise? Was my loud TV that lethal? I didn't have much time to dwell on the issue.

I continued to get tingling feelings throughout my body. So, with that, two women residents—hardly older than dating candidates for my sons, pitch that they've been ordered to do a spinal tap. Huh? I thought that was the name of a movie or something in a bar. But the real thing is creepy. Now, how many times could these "gals" have done this procedure? I dare ask and just say, "no problem." This IS a teaching hospital, btw.

So, on my side I go, knees to the chest, twist a little here and there, and one inserts a syringe in-between my vertebrae to extract some spinal fluid. The other practically closed her eyes as she appeared to be grossed-out and wanting to throw up.

Or was I imagining that?

But I gotta say, with a little local anesthetic, I would learn a lesson that would keep me sane and a good sport for all of the procedures to come. **The anticipation is worse than the procedure itself.** Thanks Lidocaine! Bring it on! (And keep a barf-bag around, just in case)

If you're claustrophobic for an MRI they have sedatives—just ask. If you're getting anxious, you're not their first—tell them. But with me flying around the hospital on gurneys all over to this exam and that, and test on test, it was already becoming quite a journey with anticipation. I could picture my Harry Potter-hair flowing in the wind, screaming down the hallways on my flying gurney, to my next cat scan, the next MRI, ultrasound...confident in my composure. I wouldn't freak-out.

But no sooner than being in my new room for another day, the reality of my whereabouts on returning from a procedure again hits, and I, forgetting where I am, cavalierly jump off the gurney only to faint and crash into my bed. Waking up and seeing my wife, I asked: "What are you doing here?" "Uh, I'm your wife?" she said, as reality was setting in. Not realizing, I also injured my shin and now officially made the "watch list." That got me another roommate—only, this one with a big eye on top that stayed quietly in a corner. It was a camera to observe my movements and to assure I, as instructed, wouldn't get out of bed. I was officially on bed arrest, and a CYA of the hospital. I named my new roommate, Mortimer.

4

This is progress?

Oh goody, a clue.

After all the bloodletting and one sample of spinal fluid and blood sent off for testing to that mystical, *Mayo Clinic* in Minnesota, something, as reported a few weeks later, showed up as being significant. I had the presence of an LGi1 antibody in my blood, and apparently, I attacked myself. At one point, as one Doctor described it, it was like a nuclear bomb went off, and now we're dealing with the aftermath and the rubble. Fuckwa! Just my luck. Now what? If I broke a leg, I would have a grasp of what was wrong with me. But what's an LGi1 antibody and is there anyone who knows what the hell to do with it? What's the minimum knowledge needed to be admitted to a hospital so as to understand the doctor speak? While they were all talking about their leukocytes and endocytes, I was more into building sites and porn sites.

Apparently, it was my immune system creating a rogue cell antibody that was the culprit. A partial explanation for my neuropathy. It attacked my own Myelin sheathing after mistaking it for a virus or some other protein. Myelin sheathing is what provides the protein protective barrier for the nerves that allows for the feelings of touch, among other things. Well, my protective barrier was basically destroyed. It's like the coating on an electrical cable that insulates the inner cables from the outside was eliminated and my electrical system is shorting itself out.

The doctors don't know how, but I had a *Bob-made,* "Pac-man" inside of me! I'm not a neurology specialist, so every time they mentioned something above my pay scale, I had trouble connecting the dots. But you gotta trust them, right? And if the doctors were baffled—where did that leave me? At first, I couldn't make heads or tails of the information, my brain befuddled and all. What happened? But with a little curiosity, tenacity and Google (who, now lives without it?), one could get a better picture, or maybe one less cloudy. Nevertheless, I was determined to get to the bottom of this story.

Hardly a secret, but that episode of fainting and falling earned me another room change—this time to the pre-ICU floor where they could monitor me a little more closely, thinking I could, also, have a heart-related issue because of the low blood pressure related passing out. An interior bed with a, surmised, drug dealer for a roommate was next to me. At least that's what my mind believed since he was on the phone, and I conjured up he was talking a lot about pot. But apparently, there are other people in the world with medical needs. How dare I think I should continue to have private rooms with a window view? I'm now in Nairobi. Nevertheless, my roommate departed the next day; alive, and in a wheelchair (this time). But I had other events, to come on my unwritten, and unfolding agenda. How does one stay in the hospital for three months?

Being in an interior bed with the surrounding curtain, as on this dreaded 6th floor, or in other words, solitary confinement, would have driven me out of my mind. I needed the outside for sure. By some good fortune, because I truly was apparently a unique case, I generally had a private room—and they always came with a window. Someone had mercy or pity on me after dealing with my squeaky wheel.

Meanwhile, for the past three weeks or so, I still can't bathe myself, or even wipe my ass without assistance. I had to be placed on some commode and get lifted by an assistant who wiped my butt, cleaned my potty, and then put everything back together again as if nothing happened. They are unpraised, brave people. All new to me, I felt embarrassed, to say the least. A little humbling. But there wasn't much of a choice unless I was going to become some shit-loaded balloon ready to burst at any moment. *That* would have been a mess. Ya think? Tending to me was like falling on a grenade. Paging TV's Mike Rowe. I've got *Dirty Jobs* for ya.

Being bedridden since my arrival to the hospital, I haven't exercised or done any of the daily routines to keep muscle. Besides, prolonged Prednisone leads to muscle wasting. My ass was practically drooping below knee-level. They keep you in bed for CYA of not falling, but muscle waste leads to the inability to get *some* exercise, to avoid waste. Kind of a Catch-22. Is falling from weakened muscles outside of bed more dangerous than weakened muscles promoted by staying *in* bed?

Because of these conflicting behaviors, without realizing it, I was becoming a vegetable—a carrot to be more precise. So, when some visitors were present, I declared that I needed some space to do my "business." They left, and the nurse set me on the commode. And when done, that's when the action started.

Apparently, while I attempted to get up, and leaning forward to pull up my sweatpants, I passed out on the bed. Picture it; pants half-pulled up, me squish on the bed, face down, splat! The nurse hit code red, blue, whatever, thinking I was breathing my last breath. So as told to me, because I'm unconscious, about half the hospital staff, after hearing the code, swarmed the room. My visitors, out in the hallway, thought they were getting a "two-fer"—a last visit AND a wake. Two for the price of one. Right out of some made for TV ER program.

A little "false alarm" as it turns out. Wipe the tears away. My fainting spells were connected in some way to whatever, still undiagnosed, illness I have. But the butt-mooning episode made me chuckle and taught me a valuable lesson.

In a hospital—there can be no modesty. And be sure there are no pimples on your hairy ass.

Hospital attire does not necessarily mandate the wearing of those open-in-the-back gowns that, you think, titillate the staff with hairy butts and banging "Daddy" balls while strolling down the halls. You don't have anything they haven't already seen enough too many times before. Depending on one's illness and convenience of examinations, you can wear any clothes that feel comfortable. But they do go psycho if you're not wearing those cute colored socks with little, white, non-slip dots on the bottoms. Obviously, so as not to slip and fall.

* * *

After another uneventful day or two, and another test or two, and a thing or two, I (with Mortimer following) would be transferred to another room. This time 3rd floor, to an outer bed with a new roommate. I heard his voice on the other side of the curtain, but where was he from, what did he look like? I could only surmise; My natural curiosity was aroused. He sounded Mideastern, but, overhearing his issues, I knew he wouldn't be a happy camper in any language. His experiencing a catheter up the you know where is not fun. Ouch!

Early on in the hospital, it was all about the news of Anthony Bourdain's suicide. So, all of his TV shows, *Parts Unknown*, (sounds like a teenage boy's expedition) were being aired. I was bewildered and sad for Anthony, but happy for the diversion to see his travelogue with food included; but I also wanted to see if there were any clues to his motive for suicide.

But it wouldn't be my lucky day, or Anthony's either. To me, nothing would be revealed. His suicide seemed like a waste. What was *his* plight? An untreatable illness like Robin Williams'? Williams' autopsy revealed Lewy Body Dementia. "My husband was trapped in the twisted architecture of his neurons and no matter what I did I could not pull him out," his wife, Susan Williams wrote:

> *"For nearly a year, in a painful odyssey that will be familiar to many patients, Williams tried to find out what was wrong with himself— and fix it. He underwent tests and scans, tried new medications, did physical therapy, worked out with a trainer, and sought out alternative treatments like self-hypnosis and yoga."*

I was, apparently, not alone in my mysterious plight, and he couldn't live with his illness or the chase.

Did they succumb to mere depression, like lots of comics with the huge fame? Or something so secret they couldn't live with it? So, I became glued to Bourdain's series in search of a clue. I watched Anthony with llamas in the mountains; driving in freezing rain with his brother at the Jersey Shore; having lunch with President Obama in Ishkaboo; among other places only Anthony Zimmern, on *Bizarre Foods*, may have dared been to before.

But if there was a clue, as to his suicide, it certainly didn't reveal itself to me. Just another show to take my mind off my major issues. Little did I realize; it was a clue to my later thinking about the same subject. Would I arrive at his same conclusion? Could I share his ultimate fate?

* * *

In this new room on the third floor, bed on the outside with a window, but on an interior courtyard, a new treatment would be tried; IVIG, intravenous applications of immunoglobulin.

Immunoglobulin: *"It is a blood product prepared from the serum of between 1,000 and 15,000 donors per batch. It gives you antibodies that your body can't make on its own so you can fight infections."* So says Google; because that's what you do when you have all of these crazy sounding diseases or treatments bandied about you and the doctors really don't have the time or inclination to explain your unknown, illness to you. But it's your body! So, you google a lot. And you want to be kept in the loop. But this IVIG would be administered to "wash out" the bad blood with some new blood contributed by the thousands along with some disease-fighting protection. Sounds almost like medieval leeches, no? Only, the equipment has been updated.

"Between 1,000 and 15,000 donors per batch" says the National Institutes of Health. That is how many people have to donate to keep treatment going for me. If I decided to be done with this, that's a lot of effort that can go elsewhere.

IVIG is always a fun experience, especially when a new nurse gets the assignment of administering their first application of a sensitive medical treatment and they're a little unsure of themselves. But oh well, who was I to complain?

Sometimes ya just gotta go with the flow, especially when you're surrounded by "gods." To doubt them would be blasphemy. Luckily, I received an intravenous application of Benadryl first to ward off any allergic reactions to the IV. That was pleasant because it made me drowsy enough to fall asleep and get through part of the hours-long ordeal. Although the first application went to five hours from the expected three, comparatively speaking, I still couldn't wipe the ole' tush... So, who was I to complain? One learns not to burn bridges with the nursing staff, so to speak, because ya never know when they'll really be needed.

But it was at this station that I would have my hair done. Just not the way one would normally think. That was when they did the EEG procedure—and this mousy looking, Bugs Bunny-type person comes to administer it. Striking up a conversation, braiding my hair with some 36 or so electrodes, she says she'll be back the next morning to do the test. No pain, she just needs to keep track of the electrical impulses given off by my brain and would need a couple of hours and maybe for me to even fall asleep. Turns out, my 'do was no better than Frankenstein's bride's hair-do.

Of course, without disappointment, Bugs showed up the next day, and proceeded to goop some gooey stuff in my hair to make contact with all 36 electrodes. THAT took an hour. And as she's finished, she then says it'll take a couple of hours and she'll return before the end of day. Well, that turned into evening, I hadn't heard from her, and the braiding was becoming a littttttttle tight. I'm not a happy A-hole. When she called the next day, of all chutzpah, I said, "if you're not here in 60 minutes, I'll rip out all the braids and maybe even kick the machine to boot." Message received—loud and clear. With that, I'm beginning to feel a little empowered.

5

Screaming Heads-in-the-Beds

As tests, meetings, and consultations proceeded, and, apparently, dwindled down the options for a diagnosis, I was then moved to the neurology, 9th floor—single room—view of Central Park, looking West! I still thought I was in heaven even though I knew I wasn't dead—sunsets 'n all. But this was hardly a consolation prize.

I even got to see the NYC Stonehenge sunset where the sun sets right between the buildings for the summer solstice at around 105th street! Not exactly to the day, but pretty close for, again, government housing! What? I can't be a little snarky? It's what colors the presence of an invisible man. "Tough titties" as my dad would say.

So here I am, the neuro-floor, just six floors removed from the last, and all of the rest of the related neuro staff.

What's changed? The TV stations don't work that well, but the morning traveling pack of the wanna-be residents still find you and make their rounds waiting for the attendant. Same hospital, just different faces. "You still here?" Some said. The goal, as the attending would say, is "to get you out of here."

One of the most peculiar exams administered was by the Neuro team. This had to be one of the most imprecise, subjective, and old-fashioned exams still being administered in our modern medical world. Fred Flintstone must have invented the procedure.

The doctor would press down on my limbs and ask for me to resist. In addition to that, he would take two index fingers, one on each side of my neck and ask while tickling me, "feel the difference?" "Huh? "Feel the difference?"

"This is modern medicine?" I asked. I couldn't see his hands, so I trusted they were his fingers... This is what precision science has come to? It had to be some outdated tradition, like so many others.

Why do we maintain 2,500-year-old traditions when, clearly, we're in an ever-changing world? This is the latest, controlled, or accurate experiment, or test, that will assist or lead to restoring my life as was known? Obviously, in the days of DNA oriented molecular biology, instant digital updates, and beyond, someone didn't get the memo to update this procedure. It felt like medieval times. They could have put leeches on me, and I wouldn't have known the difference.

The neuro floor at this point was to zero-in on what was ailing me. The liver on the way to restoration (and how was that brought about?). They had a sense of my illness and surmised that it was something nerve related causing my current malaise. But they couldn't nail the diagnosis. Was the original liver ailment really nerve related? Which came first, the chicken or the egg?

So why was I on the dreaded 9th floor: Neurology? Was it the right place to be? Maybe I should have been treated for an autoimmune abnormality which was creating the problem. Because it sounds, to me, like the autoimmune issue caused the nerve damage.

But as I heard some pieces or tried to make out what they were all talking about, I could only Google the symptoms hoping that a diagnosis would magically, materialize from the keywords.

I would learn quickly that a gazillion diagnoses would emerge but nary a few would be considered because they would have to fit into a protocol. *All* of the symptoms had to fit a specific diagnosis.

In my case, finding one specific fish in the ocean would be easier than a diagnosis.

At one point Google had me convinced I had Guillain–Barré syndrome. At least it was a name. But that would be too easy. According to the Doctors, *everything* had to fall under the classification of that illness, or it would be called something else. I went through more something-elses than "Carter's got liver pills," as they say. But a point of concern, seems like they needed a diagnosis before they would aggressively treat the affliction.

Was their treatment-toolbox big enough? Was this becoming a case of lost time? Like when one is experiencing a heart attack, Aspirin could often be immediately prescribed? Was something not done quickly enough when neuropathy was in the picture? Or was I just a stubborn-to-diagnose case and they were in over their heads insisting they first have a name in the interest of, once again, covering their butts? Maybe. Regardless, I'm thinking, what would be the downside to err on the side of aggressively administering something as harmless as an Aspirin when it's apparently known that early neuropathy can, sometimes, be arrested with early aggressive treatment. And it wasn't a secret that I had neuropathy! So why wasn't I given a choice as to whether I wanted to stay in Mt. Sinai or be transferred to a more suitable facility that was more equipped and staffed to handle my case?

The room overlooking Central Park, number 904 West, was like being at The Plaza Hotel, so to speak. But there were also screamers. Some are moaners crying out in pain or wanting attention. Some could be pre-death, so I heard, but others were on a more regular cycle of measured cries—the Encephalitis screamers. All day long, unless they were sedated, they would scream on a regular basis at the top of their lungs. Sad, really. I was told they either don't know what they're doing or know where they are. I asked my doctor:" Are they trapped crying for help but couldn't receive it—they're unconscious?"

But being someone with a body affliction such as mine, it occurred to me, now, full of fear, that I was a small distance from tipping over to being in the same condition—a screaming Head-in-the-Bed. No, No, No!!! I feel like I'm in Dr. Seuss's "Green Eggs and Ham." I am a head on a body, a head on a company, a head that's fed. But I will not be a Head-in-the-Bed, I will not.

No one can do anything for those people at that point. You can't terminate their lives. Euthanasia or mercy killing is not allowed. It's against the law!

Someone should be prepared ahead of time for this possible outcome. Why should I have to be reactive instead of being proactive? Like an emergency ripcord on a failing parachute? Like a whispered, prenuptial agreement? Or a spy's Cyanide pill? Just in case. I don't want to be the shmuck that waits too long.

But how does one start thinking about such things? How does one have a civil conversation about it with others? "Sure Bob, we're all lining up to see who'll first push you over the edge."

And if you believe my brain was scrambled, what could that mean for all the other people in my life? Could I wake up one day with a frozen body only to realize I'm just as mobile and aware as a head of cabbage with eyes? And all, while no one is willing or able to put me out of my misery.

All I could do was to be a good sport and take whatever was dished out by my godly doctor team. My Neuro doctor, a nice guy, but a little wormy and old, who was in touch with his "colleague" at the Mayo Clinic, insisted that a biopsy of the ankle-nerve and the thigh muscle was necessary to help determine the cause and extent of the neuropathy. Only, the procedure had to be scheduled with a certain doctor because *my* doctor trusted him. But why were *"we"* relying on a colleague? The mention of Mayo was impressive; but was my condition out of *my* doctor's league? Who would tell?

Two weeks go by before he's even able to get in touch with the other doctor. "Oh, sorry, been on vacation. We'll schedule for next week." Or so he said. Imagine? Hotel Mt. Saini is charging a humongous daily rate for the private room I'm occupying while we're on the runway and some other doctor is on vacation. But I forget, Medicare picks up the bill. Although the procedure was easy enough to complete: a snip here, a cut and some stitches there, getting the results was another story. After three more weeks we still didn't have the full report. Oh, and by the way, when they snipped the nerves in the foot and thigh, I will have a permanent lack of feeling in those areas, forever, so they said! Ya gotta love those "Oh, by the ways..."

All the while there were ever more tests, more MRI's, EKG's, Cat scans, etc. The list was endless because all the doctors had afterthoughts since there was still no clear diagnosis. So, let's just do another test for the heck of it. They were on a noble mission to heal, or that's what we choose to believe.

They didn't seem to care because, apparently to the medical bunch, money is no object. They own the equipment. So, it was like owning an ice-cream maker; "let's just have some ice-cream" and bill the insurance company! We're still playing Medical, "Whack-a-Mole," Bob!

Yet, nothing fit into a neat little identification box. Just dutifully do any and all tests while attempting to complete the puzzle and see what picture we're left with.

Nice that I've aroused their intellectual curiosity, but the solution to that puzzle would continue to prove somewhat elusive. And maybe the answer isn't in the form they're looking for or even exists.

Nevertheless, they continue to bill for their time. I can't blame greed entirely on the doctors, they're part of the system.

Even though their Hippocratic Oath demands healing first; because of their liability, their incentive to protect their own asses becomes a conflict of interest. So, they over test, administer needless procedures, and over medicate, leading to unnecessary expenses that enrich the doctors and the entire healthcare system. Talk about a conflict of interest. Who is on this watch? Is there a "fox minding the chickens?"

Every day it was practically something else. What would they reveal or not reveal? What fun ride would we do today? Just bill Uncle Sam or the insurance companies. The more the merrier in an uncontested, "for-profit" scenario. That's "Time and material" in the construction business. Something to always be wary of since there's no fixed cost and therefore nothing to stop overrunning budgets. Just keep billing.

But thanks to Medicare...

To be fair, with my spaghetti bowl of issues and symptoms, ruling out or confirming whether it was a linguini, or a fettuccine, to my doctors, was, apparently, necessary. They can't make a diagnosis if one component of the disease doesn't fit the established description of the disease and therefore, previously prescribed medication. Ya can't call it a Lasagna if it's made with Spaghetti noodles! Yet, the money-meter ticking on this illness was non-stop. Talk about aggressive procedures of monopolistic healthcare providers. That's their business model. Just keep on billing.

At the end of the day it was determined, absent that rogue-cell doing the damage, I was a healthy guy—just an ex-homebuilder moving on with life. The "atomic bomb exploded, it's now a sunny day after, and we're dealing with the mess." Oh contraire!

No cancer, tumors, major blood deficiencies, nothing for now, except the bewildering presence of neuropathy, caused by what?

So, meantime, early on, the bilirubin was the liver number of the day. We all observed and followed the decrease in the number like it was a countdown or a horse race. It was more than 10 at the beginning of this ordeal, making me a candidate for a transplant. Normal is supposed to be below 1. So, every day it was watched like a stock ticker. Only, I was "short selling" bilirubin. Eventually, with the prescribed medication and the discontinuance of the Augmentin, the number came down, obviating the need for a transplant—whew! But was there a definitive reason for the acute liver failure? And why, all of a sudden, after 69 years of my liver performing just fine, did I come up with liver failure anyway?!

But...hidden deep somewhere in the Google annals of my laptop...

" *From: FDA.gov... "AUGMENTIN XR should be used only* " *to treat or prevent infections that are proven or strongly suspected to be caused by bacteria." (GlaxoSmithKline 2006)*

And from: The National Institutes of Health "LiverTox": "Amoxicillin-clavulanate is currently the most common cause of clinically apparent, drug induced acute liver injury both in the United States and Europe."

(Evans J, Hannoodee M., et. al)

AUGMENTIN XR is another name for Amoxicillin-clavulanate.

The pulmonologist said I had a VIRUS! Why was I given an antibacterial drug?! Repetitively!!

Well, if the irresponsible usage of Augmentin wasn't the cause of my liver failure, what was? That I had a fetish for ice-cream?

What was the obvious change in my lifestyle, other than taking Augmentin, that could affect my liver?! The virus? And imagine if I didn't have the wits to stop the Augmentin, or the hospital unnecessarily removed my liver! What other chains of gob-smacked catastrophic events might have ensued?

So, what was everything else about? What, then, was creating the neuropathy?

It remains to this day, the connection the doctors can't or won't make—hiding under cover of "idiopathic." All I know is that with the Augmentin overdose and abuse, and the subsequent or concomitant liver failure, and the immediately invading neuropathy, there were so many *ands*, all occurring about the same time. That's connection enough to come to my own conclusions. Over-the-top circumstantial and coincidental evidence—but you can't convict?

If it walked like a duck and acted like one—to me, it is a duck. It was too coincidental to be otherwise. But when confronted with my theory, no doctor would commit because obviously the science is still out of reach compared to diagnosing a "cold."

There is a Patient's Bill of Rights, you know. And they're posted all over a hospital. You can refuse tests, treatment, anything you want. But remember, it's at your own peril. Being a patient, one takes on risks doubting their physicians. After all, we entrust them with our lives as they're more empowered, not to mention, we believe, more qualified, than us. Or so we've been led to believe.

But gods they're not. So, ask questions!

But what stops them from playing the "idiopathic" game for the sake of Cover-Ya-Ass? They do make mistakes just like any other profession. They're human. But some get carried away thinking their years of education make them infallible and all-knowing. And that's why there's medical malpractice insurance. Someone's malpracticing. Why do we have the gall to shield them from irresponsible behavior by limiting lawsuits? Do we just rationalize all improprieties that "shit happens?" I don't think any system is 100% infallible. Think about the "unsinkable" Titanic; the birth defects from the Thalidomide pill; turning down J.K. Rowling's *Harry Potter*; filling the Hindenburg with hydrogen.

"Shit happens?"

6

And the beat goes on...

Meanwhile, my neuro doctor thinks he has a handle on what my problem is but notices that I'm in no physical shape to address the world. He believes physical therapy would be in order before discharge. And the best way to accomplish that will be for me to be rehabbed as part of the hospital stay. So, down to the 2nd floor we go—the rehab floor. Yet, if I recall, I think he was biding time. But why?

So, I would be there for three more weeks. Two at first, and an extended week for "good behavior." "Then, I would go home—right?" I must say, it did wonders for my strength and rehab of my mental outlook. Things looked encouraging. I was able to wipe myself and shower alone again. I could only think of an old Jackie Gleason, *Honeymooner's* skit: "Alice—look out, vavavavooom and away we goooo!"

The rehab floor was probably the most positive experience. I had my laptop, my recipes, and workouts six times a week for a total of 3 1/2 hours a day. It was all split into two sessions, mornings and the afternoon following LUNCH! I had my TV food shows, ice cream, and shortbread cookies. I had the equivalent of a continuous wait-staff. What could be better?

They asked how often I wanted to come, per week, to occupational and physical therapy. I said, "I want out—how often do I need?"

Yet with all the comforts of a hotel stay in a hospital, I was beginning to get used to the lifestyle of this stay. Sort of like a Stockholm Syndrome captive, I guess. But I entered this hospital because I was under the impression I was going to get better. Reason for optimism would be justified. Although I could understand their cautiousness. No one would commit to: "You'll experience good health in 36 days, 10 hours, and 21 minutes." This is the CYA capital of the modern world. No one is going to commit and stick their necks out!

Frequently trying to break the monotony, I became the Jack Nicholson-type from *One Flew Over the Cuckoo's Nest*. I was the one, who, instead of rolling the ball back to my therapist, would roll the ball in another direction across the room to bounce off a wall, just to see if there was another life-form in the same room. A little disruptive, perhaps. Inconsequential fun. It got a few giggles from the not-quite-dead crowd.

Being among the rehab residents could also be depressing. And I was part of it, low blood pressure and all. I probably looked pretty bad myself, and sad, so much so that the personnel followed me around with a chair in case of dizziness, which happened a few times.

But there were other cases that looked worse. Some with helmets, heads leaning, almost comatose-looking patients. They went through the motions on some path to recovery.

How did I have a right to protest in light of their plight. Like the cliché: "There but for the grace of God, go I."

Though, that might not be as bad a trade as on first glance. I might trade you six months of looking and acting like a vegetable for one, full-body neuropathy, to last maybe a lifetime?

Yet it all seemed like a nightmare. What was I doing here and when will it be over?

One rehab doctor tritely proffered, "You'll look back on this like a bad dream." Which might have been convincing if he wasn't so focused on banging the snot-nosed resident who wouldn't leave his side.

I still thought I was really in some B movie or dreamland, and it would all get better; never realizing that the medical team was also struggling for a diagnosis and treatment.

Then there was the party and a real reality check! The young candy stripers would come around every day trying to enlist participation in some social event to rouse the patients. You know, like meet your favorite pet, finger painting for fun (you know what that looked like.), or we're watching a movie today, *Fred McMurray's, the Nutty Professor*.

Hey! I'm not one of those old, gray-haired, people, head shlunked down, with an illness in need of a "G" rated movie. I remember, as a young boy, 65 years ago, people lined up in their wheelchairs on the Long Beach, N.Y. boardwalk; "Nursing Home Alley." They looked and moved like bumper cars at an amusement park. But I'm going to be healthy again one day and resume my macho, builder's life. Right?

But party-day, or the party-day I would participate was cake-day downstairs in the social room. Nothing like being in a room where you get to be surrounded by the Grace-of-God crew. I felt I still didn't fit in with them.

WHAT WAS I DOING THERE? I thought I was on the path to recovery. But, to me, this was something out of a horror movie. What are they looking at or planning to do with this head in a wheelchair? Did they all know something I didn't? Like that *Twilight Zone* episode "Eye of the Beholder," when all were treating a beautiful girl and they were perplexed at how to solve her problem when it was revealed that *everyone else had pig noses*!

Eventually they needed my suite for a paying guest. So, I, once again, got reassigned. They would move me down the hall for the last few days until it was decided that I would undergo Plasma exchange.

They're really doing some weird shit to me—Plasma exchange, bodily fluid transfers...Is any poo sticking to the wall, or are we chimps with our hair on fire just flailing our arms?

Roommate on the inside—window to my left, on the outside. Roommates in the hospital, I've found, are not really that sociable, so don't look for a new buddy so fast. They have their own issues and pain—not to mention visitors, phone calls, sleep, bathroom noises, language barriers, and moaning. Don't get the idea people are any more interested in the outer-space stuff that's being done to you than you are more than a fleeting moment interested in them. They're not coming to your rescue!

Maybe I wasn't going home at the end of therapy. I remember chatting with someone at the nurse's station at 1:30 a.m. with an anxiety attack about my perceived difficulty of breathing. With my constricted torso, sometimes my lungs can't get a full breath of air. Nice thought.

I was doing fine under the circumstances, up until this point. But I think the reality of it all was maybe getting to me. Why would I even think of such an anxiety provoking situation? Maybe the wormy doctor's prompt that he can give me something for *it* aroused my subconscious. (He's a neuro doc; he should know.) Maybe he knew what would follow in my case but wasn't revealing it to me. Or more precisely, I suspect, he didn't really have a clue. The *Twilight Zone* theme music now pervades my head along with some dancing, body-snatching, pods and Mick Jagger music.

Now, here's the thing. Since they "narrowed" down my diagnosis to *idiopathic, autoimmune induced, neuropathy*; now they want to administer a regime of blood change in the form of Plasmapheresis.

"Plasmapheresis, or plasma exchange, is a procedure which involves the removal, treatment, and return of blood to the body to remove antibodies, thereby preventing them from attacking their targets. This blood purification procedure is used to treat several autoimmune diseases." (Patients-LikeMe)

Google again. More poo on the wall, because they don't have a diagnosis—let alone a cure. So, they insert an IV in your arm and you stay in bed for about 3-4 hours while they spin your blood through a machine to filter out the bad blood, presumably including the rogue antibodies. Needless to say—I didn't feel any different afterward. For that matter, they could have prescribed prune juice as a cure.

We're all still playing Helen Keller, groping in the dark.

With this new development, before the rest of the doses, we have *another* conversation about *another* required procedure. I'm told this time that in order to administer the plasmapheresis, on a more regular basis, they need to insert a 1/8-1/4" IV in my neck to handle the greater volume of blood. Note to self: Riiiiight—IV in my neck.

So, the next morning, down to the operating room, I go for an incision to be made in my neck-vein and a tube inserted, in same, to receive the plasma exchange. They call it a "port." For two weeks more, the IV stayed there. You know, the car commercial with the black dude and this little head, his conscience, telling him what to do? Me and my new little friend (named *Wilsomina* after Tom Hank's "Wilson") sticking out of my neck while I'm walking my instructed

30 laps around the nurse's station, for exercise, with my walker. My trusting "friend," *Wilsomina*, paraded around, would be there to receive the plasma for my medical procedure that, otherwise, would not have been able to be administered.

After about seven sessions, and two weeks later, other than making a new friend, and me, again, saying I didn't notice any difference, I think the last person in the hospital gave up. Another white flag. Hadn't they ever seen a case such as mine? Aside from refusing the permanent adoption of my newfound companion, I was going to go home shortly, sans my Wilsomina. We had to break up.

As we parted ways, neither of us overtly, lamenting our separation, they withdrew the catheter from my neck, watched my status for the next day, and by mid-August, said, "ba-bye."

7

Ob-la-di Ob-la-da, Life Goes On

Nine rooms—in twelve weeks.

That's more than the number of rooms I occupied going on vacations in the last five years!! At least half of my rooms in the hospital were private. Almost all of them put me next to the window when shared. Toward the end of my hospital incarceration, I think everyone who was responsible for room selection felt pity for my situation and for my sanity. So, they, per my request, gave me privacy, and considered the window paramount. Three months was a long time to be confined with no end in sight and only being able to access fresh air from the outside of the hospital for an hour.

When the cleanup staff would enter the room, unannounced and on their own time, always proved disruptive, regardless of whether you were sleeping or doing some other activity. Always changing the bedding, cleaning the garbage pails, sweeping, mopping, or dusting the floors. Between that and the food-order person, pill administration, nurses, doctors, administrative staff, tests, and all the rest, it's probably more restful to be homeless and sleep in Grand Central Station.

Breakfast would actually be the highlight of my day. But three months is also a long time to rarely get my breakfast order right.

First of all, for just about my whole life, breakfast was an anathema to me. Skipped it until lunchtime—but I was certainly hungry by then.

By the time 7:30a.m. came around, in the hospital, I was practically growling. The steroids only made it worse. Don't delay a hungry prednisone user without expecting to hear the feedback. So, while the anticipation was great before receiving my feast, the disappointment was so much worse when they didn't deliver all that was ordered and anticipated.

Irritating to say the least, but it was certainly accentuated by the steroids. My short fuse was always ready to be lit! Too frequently I felt like I got some guy's breakfast from down the hall. Hope he liked *my* order. But it's not rocket science to get the right order delivered.

Now, I miss those days of anticipating a morning breakfast. So, it was continued when I came home from the hospital: bowls of semolina, farina, grits, all with butter, milk, maple syrup, nuts, or honey. All starting at 4a.m. because of the Prednisone. But I love honey.

It's something that makes my day, as nothing else does except maybe peanut butter and my wife Dee.

8

Me and Dee

I remember when Dee and I had our first date.

It was a blind one arranged by her cousin.

We talked on the phone as two eager people fantasizing in the sexiest way about what the other sounded or looked like. But I had been so disappointed with blind dates that I came prepared for our first meeting. As she opened the door, I greeted her wearing Groucho Marx glasses along with his eyebrows and a big nose, just in case.

You can speculate what my "in-case" intentions were. Yes, I was disguised. But, when the door opened, my expectations were not disappointed—my search would be over. My balls rang in my head.

I had to put my foot in the door to prevent her from closing it and assured her I had no nefarious intentions. I immediately took off the disguise and revealed my true ugly self—not really.

We had dinner that night sharing an artichoke at a local Italian restaurant in NYC's "Village." It would be beyond true love at first sight when a couple slurps the petals and sauce off of their fingers from a stuffed artichoke on their first date.

I felt like my teenage hero, Albert Finney, from the eating scene in the movie, *Tom Jones*. So, the next night we were together, I got up the courage and asked her, under my breath, to marry me. And a little louder, I also asked if she liked peanut butter. She said, "yes," so, I knew our lives, from that point on, would change forever. I love peanut butter.

We met in early Summer when I was 36 and she was 26. Blissfully we traveled to California that August for an end of summer road trip down the Pacific Coast Highway, route 1, from SF to LA, stopping along the way to notable tourist attractions of Big Sur, The Hearst Castle, and Harmony, CA, just to name a few. I told her she was fun to travel with as we proceeded south on the outside of the road-way—with no guardrail. If I were any more nervous on the drive, for fear of heights, I could have easily gone over the edge.

It was on the trip that while in the motel room one morning, Dee was greeted, as she came out of the shower, with a diamond en-gagement ring on the washing counter. Yes, I had it in my pocket on the way out on the plane. Of course, she was shocked, said yes, and felt compelled to immediately tell the world; namely her family. But before we have all these salivating family members on both coasts burning up the phone lines, I said, "Let's keep it our secret until we return." She did tell "Fred from Fresno" in the parking lot though. A stranger satisfied her need to tell *someone*. But little could I foresee the road trip to come.

We were engaged three months after we met and married within six altogether—before she turned 27. And noooo, it was not a shot-gun wedding. I was just head over heels about her and felt the music had stopped for my dating and it was time to settle down and move on. Why delay. And on such short notice to find a wedding site, turned out, that coming Thanksgiving weekend was available, and with that, off on a Honeymoon in Rio.

Fast forward thirty something years later in the hospital and I'm eating the bland cooking of hospital chefs.

After three months of having a roasted, oregano-spiced, chicken leg and thigh, for dinner, with mashed potatoes and whole kernel corn—practically every day, because little else appeared to be edible, my staple diet became double ice cream, double cookies, apple juice, and who knows what other Prednisone induced carbohydrate cravings that needed satiating. Obviously, the chicken and mashed potatoes were the appetizer. All that followed or mattered, to me, was the main course. I C E C R E A M!!!! Hey—at a dosage of 70mgs a day, the dessert craving is irresistible. I dare you, but not for real. I even had to make friends with the food delivery guy to take care of my needs—for a price, of course. I had the candy treats, for the offering, which he didn't have access to, for the trade. But I was a certified, Prednisone, junkie-slave—and all legal!

At least the ice cream for lunch and dinner was comforting; today vanilla for lunch, chocolate for dinner. Yum. At this rate, they could cut my leg off in pursuit of a diagnosis because the ice-cream would make it all better.

Yet, I was still living in some nightmare from which I was under the impression I would soon awake.

9

Always thinking of business

Now, my restaurant kitchen is like a small cockpit. It takes one to fly it. If a second person is there it's only to take over in case the first one drops dead. Someone has to put out the lights. But it's designed that way as a business model. So, if an employee doesn't show up, that could be a problem. That's the downside or my Achilles' Heel. That's why it's designed as an owner-operated shop. Owners show up! Unless you're in the hospital, like me! Until I make the employee an offer he can't refuse, I'll remain on edge for the days he doesn't show on time, or even comes at all. But gaining notoriety for the restaurant was always paramount.

Just prior to entering the hospital, Smoked was invited to participate in a BBQ cook-off. Mind you, it was my first venture into competition with Smoked. But on top of an invitation from the competition promoter, I was driven or encouraged by our rave reviews and even an excellent Yelp rating.

We were competing, albeit on a local level, but some of the biggest, award-winning smokehouses from the N.Y.C metropolitan area were entered. It was exciting.

Some had their usual fare and entered for the exposure. Others even came armed with all their trophies to display; and one with a smoked whole hog laying regally on the table as if sunning itself and saying, "I am all that pig. Dare to compete with me?"

Modestly, I produced my usual presentation: a couple of slices of my tasty brisket, my smoked baked beans in a cup, and a wedge of freshly sliced Cara Cara orange for taste, color, and the Italian way of cleansing the palate between courses.

Apparently, Smoked had been flying under the radar for the past two years and the competition was taken by surprise. There was some commotion between the judges, and they took a little longer than all contestants had, anxiously, expected, until finally a verdict was revealed. Smoked would be the winner of the 2018 North Regional BBQ Showdown, winning for best Brisket. And "Bob the Builder," author, now restaurateur, even winning over an Iron Chef competitor, was champ for the year. The pig was knocked out. It would be my last contest, though, not realizing my ordeal to follow, and I was happy to go out on top. Jerry Seinfeld and I would have another something in common.

Now, armed with confidence and some optimism, my plan while in the hospital to increase revenues was to fill the early morning and lunchtime time slots with breakfast and brunch maintaining the brand. Grits 'n sausage, smoked bacon wrapped plantains, baking corn muffins, and other traditional Southern fare. I would use the time productively and to keep myself busy in the process. I may end up with a droopy ass, but at least I could occupy my mind and have something to show for my incarceration. Hey, I suppose if I were in jail—which I sort-of was—this is what it would look like. So, we bought a cheap laptop and a printer to pass the time.

I was going to research all my recipes and assemble them into a compendium of Bob's "Smoked" Recipe Book for the store. Turns out the printer was a bad idea because it became cumbersome with the paper and space, and I could easily save all the recipes to email and print them later. But, nevertheless, it was a plan that kept me occupied. Where else was I going while trapped in my time warp?

10

The Gas Scam and Fart Food

Fortunately, the catering started picking up around holiday time. Orders were coming in for up to 350 people per week and the cooking time could start as early as 5a.m. for orders due in the city by 11a.m.

Without realizing it for a while, this *was* filling up my morning time slot, making the complicated breakfast and brunch idea, contemplated to fill that time, unnecessary. Scheduling the catering activities and keeping me busy was wonderful. Although local doctor-testing and physical therapy sessions sometimes created conflicts, it was keeping me busy and the mind off of my other issues. The only problem with this was the increased anxiety or worries created by either the Prednisone and or the illness. Will the help come in on time? Will they schedule the order properly? Will they arrive on time at their destination; and just about everything else under the sun?

While in the hospital, the dizzying schedule for Dee and the rest of the family was another thing I had to think about. Back and forth to the hospital from NJ to NYC, parking, where to stay, the store, the bills for the store and home, the help, among other things, and me. It wasn't a two-person partnership, anymore, with me pulling my load.

It was all overwhelming for her. I may be challenging on a good day. But with my own OCD for business on top of this...?

And what did I know or feel? It was, in my mind, all about me, not realizing the toll it was taking on the rest of the family having to deal with the illness mixed in with the emotions. I was the one with the problem. But before they came in or after they left the room, I had NO idea what stresses they were lugging around or had to deal with. They were just more or less out of sight.

But things eventually catch up in one way or another. In retrospect I feel badly that we *can* get blindly consumed. But excuse me, and sorry. This is where the "fire" was.

When Dee came on a warm, late side of a summer Friday afternoon to visit in the hospital, she remarked about a call from the utility company demanding payment for a past-due bill in the amount of $1,500 or they were going to shut off service immediately.

Shutting off electric service to an ongoing restaurant business is practically a death sentence. And clearer heads would not prevail.

Although somewhat fishy sounding, I play a cash management game every month: "Rob Peter to pay Paul" and all that. I don't like it, but this is what my restaurant world has come down to. Probably not much different than so many other people in the country trying to make ends meet.

So maybe the shut-off call was real. I certainly wasn't in the frame of mind to verify the story, especially with my head mesmerized with the sunset view overlooking Central Park.

The caller to Dee demanded a debit card payment be delivered to an unknown account. So, she disappears on some ridiculous mission, on this hot-summer Friday after work, to deliver payment before the "shutoff."

After going to a store to buy a debit card, the bank, and make some phone calls, my "*Gone with the Wind's*, *Scarlett O'Hara* paid.

Never was the caller to be traced or heard from again.

Bottom line, as confirmed by the police, it was a scam. I felt frustrated and helpless in my predicament that I was unable of preventing the situation. Ultimately, my store, my dream. I was, now, practically, incapable of protecting my family.

When illness is around—it's not really the time to be doing business. But what were the choices? In saner times I doubt I would have been inclined to succumb to the demand. But how can a guy think when he can't even wipe his own ass? I'm sure Dee was doing the best she could while being consumed by the tsunami of misery around her!

Just another reason to feel inadequate in relation to the bargain we made when we got married. And I may sound sexist, believing only I could handle this among other issues, but I'm not the same as when we "contracted," some 35 years ago, to live together, "'till death do us part," for the rest of our lives. Granted, nothing stays the same over the years, and partners "grow old" together. But does it also imply that one of us is entitled to drastically be in need and it's a "roll of the dice" as to who gets the designation of "Caregiver?" Maybe I'd like to die on my sword and not demand, that at some point, my wife and family be mandated and trapped to also endure my torture. On the other hand; "In sickness ...'till death do us part?"

It was all so sudden. I hadn't had the faintest clue that the game-plan, I envisioned for my life and family, would take an unexpected turn. As a guy I was expected to provide for those I loved most. OK, dreamus interruptus. Now what? Although my immediate response was to "jump ship," and bail, I figured I'd buy some time and rather than panic—let's see what comes of the whole thing. Maybe we have a chance to "reboot."

* * *

Prednisone, a hungry hombre, and food recipes? That's not a prescription to lose weight. At this point I was gaining on *Star Wars'* Jabba the Hutt. My belly had a mind of its own and slowly creeped. Getting bigger, and bigger, I felt if I had one more bite, my belly would explode. I doubt Jabba ever worried about that! But heeeeeey-eeeee, there's always room for more when Prednisone is your friend and on your side.

So, another one of the diversionary highlights of my hospital stay was TV's, *Diners, Drive-ins, and Dives,* with Guy Fieri. Gotta say, he *is* cookie cutter programming right down to his canned remarks. Although I rarely watched while home, the show was something to look forward to; greasy, fart-loaded recipes 'n all. It was usually on the weekends in the evening, so, while in the hospital, I really looked forward to it because his show filled the quiet weekends with entertainment and imagined supersonic farts (Eddie Murphy's Hercules?). I mean, if all the hospital wannabes and doctors were off, who was going to keep me busy? Yet, although I wasn't previously a big fan of his, he was some sort of a treat because he went to dozens of restaurants across the country sampling chef's creations. (Funny how every restaurant he went to was always crowded. Odd.) I was, then, able to see who's making and who's eating what. And then, his BBQ stops were also special. Other ideas abounded, especially how could I tweak or integrate some of the foods we were making into the recipes on this show or vice versa? Nevertheless, it took my mind off of things and kept me occupied while googling away. Of course, there was always Anthony Zimmern's show...But that had a little more historical, travelogue feel to it, so it was only a supplement to the urchin-haired, Fieri's show.

With my voracious appetite, another one of the side effects of the Prednisone, was that while reviewing recipes they all looked delicious!

I wanted this one! I wanted that one! And, to make and eat them all! Like a kid in a candy shop, without the calories or a mom to run interference!

So, I ended up with more than 1,000 recipes and a stack of paper 12 inches high! Think about it, though, what was I going to do with 1,000 recipes? I would have to, eventually, weed them out. But Prednisone made me a hungry slave to those recipes! That's a diet, for ya, for losing weight. You're so busy finding and editing recipes, who has time to eat?!

One doctor did comment about the effects of a sustained Prednisone, induced, diet, "The belly goes "Pop! And it's tough to lose." Now, look at me. I can't see below my waist. But the way things were going, who had to or what was I missing?

And all the while, and not to forget, another effect of the illness, a peculiar smell pervades my nose, all the time. It's weird—I can't describe it. It's sometimes sweet, musty, smoky, dentist's office, whatever; but unclassifiable and variable. Nevertheless, seeing it has a connection to the ole' factory nerve, that seems to be the new keyword—*Nerve*. Now, my nose competes with my dog's for weird smells.

11

Mov'n on Again with Memories

Remember the trite doctor who said I'll probably look back on this in a couple of years like a bad dream?

To which I, now, say, "Maybe I don't want to wake up." I look at others and ask: "Am I supposed to measure against them as some litmus test?"

It was the other way around once. Up until the day I went into the hospital, I was basically, "Mission Accomplished." I didn't expect much. My life's top priorities WERE accomplished. I finished my test early, put my pencil down, but was denied the pleasure to then go out and play.

Do I, now, need the pain of climbing an unrequested mountain? How much time is there remaining in my life to climb that mountain—and at what cost?

So, just about 12 weeks after being transferred to NYC, I was sent home to the prospects of home-healthcare and the end of a summer that I never saw start. But before going home, we had a stop to make.

I had located the manufacturer of a favorite puff-pastry right in the South Bronx, just a couple of miles from the hospital. Of course, we had to stop. You're in the neighborhood and you don't drop in? Besides, I welcomed the distraction of leaving the hospital. Once again, my mind tried to return to "normal." Let's get back to "life." Use detours and time productively.

The best puff-pastry is made with butter. This was no less. If it has vegetable shortening but doesn't have butter, it can't be as good—no fat, no taste.

The detour to the Bronx reminded me of when we were in Tuscany, Italy. Oh, why not just drive a few hundred miles to Pisa and then Milan to see Leonardo da Vinci's, *The Last Supper*. Turns out, it was little more than a painting on a deteriorating war-torn wall. But hey—we were "in the neighborhood." I've traveled that way wherever we go. What's of interest close by? Visiting becomes all part of the adventure.

The doctor who described the situation as a nuclear bomb going off and, now we're dealing with the aftermath—the reconstruction. Well, even Hiroshima rebuilt, although maybe in several thousand days—and we're only on day 276 here. But is this the reconstruction of Hiroshima, or is it after Hurricane Maria, Puerto Rico; reconstruction-style tossing paper-towel rolls; relegated to a stepchild?

In that case I have some serious choices to make. I don't see how this can go on forever unless I have a compelling distraction to take my mind off of things. Like the restaurant which had begun to look promising, sales wise. Or maybe something else.

I also remain optimistic for my recovery, if I can last long enough. But maybe I'm also just being a wishful thinker, ignorant, and naive. I'm the experiment.

* * *

While in the hospital, the restaurant always lurked in my mind. It was my plan that I would get through this thing, get better, then return to the store. That was my "hope" or optimism that I would get better, my reason for trusting "the system." I was going to hit the ground running by planning ahead for the things I felt the restaurant needed to survive and prosper. There had to be a revised business model that would work. But what was my optimism based on?

So, after getting home from the hospital and culling some recipes, I started interviewing for help with the kitchen, breakfast, and baking detail. It would be difficult finding that specific type of chef. Some accepted and applied, but others failed to show for the interview.

A realistic dream, perhaps, but not to happen. For one thing the talent pool in the restaurant business is not known for many positive things. Flexibility is not a well-known trait. On top of that, my bodily carnage is overwhelming, especially at my age and stage. I lack the energy and oomph to see it all through.

Six months after leaving Mt. Saini, I'm still entertaining thoughts about terminating my life. My Suicidal ideation: "thinking about it," is much closer to ways of thinking that are accepted in the non-Abrahamic; Judeo, Christian, Islamic religious traditions. According to the Hindu and Jain religions, it's called Prayopavesa and Santhara respectively, a non-violent death from starvation.

I'm a Boomer with three marvelous boys grown to men. All established, on their way in life. And, obviously, all are not happy with my thoughts about self- termination. Regardless that I've outlived my usefulness and they have the independence that I can be more of an annoyance to them than a pleasure or necessity. Do I have to be that marginalized because it's difficult for my children to spend time with me and it's painful for them to see their dad failing? I don't want to be that last leaf on a tree after the nuclear winter.

They've even offered to pay for our expenses for the rest of their parent's lives. Good men, I love their response. But a new paradigm of taking care of mom and dad? I would never contemplate such a tax on my children; another loan to pay just when they're starting out? It made me pause for my thoughts! That's part of the obsession with making SMOKED succeed. I don't want to have to rely on my children for financial support. But if healthcare is not available to all, perhaps from early on, a different system for healthcare should be instituted.

After all the time, encouragement, money, and love invested in them—maybe it's not such a bad "business" plan for them to reciprocate. Diversified investments in three children and a wife. Take note future moms and dads: Invest a lot of love and as much opportunity, as you can, in your children. Maybe it'll be an unintended extra component and return on your investment in child-rearing. Although they may hear you and not let you know, be aware when you've overstayed the party.

* * *

Now, every morning when opening my eyes (talk about hopeful), I wiggle my toes. Neuropathy still there? I wiggle my fingers. Numbness still there? And lying in bed motionless is like being in a turtle's shell until I try to move, and I realize I'm banging against my shell. I don't quite feel the constriction. But every morning rising out of bed, I try to lift the weight of my invisible armor from around my chest, that constant bear-hug of the gut; the compression sock feeling from the hands up to the elbows and to the armpits; the puffy blown-up toes and feet, up to the thighs; the tight-fitting, body-vest up to the neck—it's all still there. And that's before I get out of the bed and deal with all the rest of this curse. So, if you get bored with hearing about it during this book, then, and maybe only then, will you have an inkling of how I feel, 24/7. Yes, my plight, like crawling across a desert, has now been shared with you, the reader. And with our mouths open, they're both full of sand. Only, not forever. Your agony here will one day be over; certainly, sooner than mine...

Is this what I want to live with for the rest of my life?

Would you?

Oh, but you'll say you don't have the affliction. You can't answer. Well, it wasn't very long ago that I didn't either; and I don't want to live with it! But I don't even know how I continue.

Some say, what about all the people who have afflictions or illnesses since early-on in their lives? I say they've learned to adapt; to grow with their illness from a younger age. It has defined their reality for so long that everything they learned already took that into account. In reality, although I can't speak for them, and it's presumptuous, for sure. But this is what their life has been and is to them.

Maybe they have young children whom they'd like to contribute to their growth and development. And some of them, like in the case of Stephen Hawking, the theoretical physicist, he had a brain far more contributing to society than mine. But he still had a purpose.

When people persistently offer books on yoga and mindfulness to challenge my wadabouts, I say, how about reading the 1000-word article from *The NY Times* about "A Debate Over Rational Suicide" and then, maybe I'll read 1000 words of your book. This is my life. Why do others get to control it if I'm of no threat to them? As a matter of fact, I'm the Patriot. I'm not wasting taxpayer's money to stay alive with frivolous expenditures paid by the state toward a fruitless end.

I had a doctor who told me about fracturing his shoulder and his arm from falling off of a horse and said I should be grateful for the extent of my illness, comparatively speaking. Really? Like Doc, I'm in a straight-jacket made of errant nerves and muscle, maybe for the rest of my life, and you're equating my torture with your broken arm in a cast? A few assistant's eyes rolled after hearing his remark. Really Doc?

I remember my mother used to walk the same way I do now. Like on stumps, walking like a penguin, unbalanced gait. Gravity slowly winning the fight. Although I never really paid attention to her non-hospitalized, ailments, it seems to me, I have a lot of what she had.

But our parents talked about very little in the interest of protecting us. Like the mysterious cousin we all whispered about who had cancer (shhh).

Then, there was my mother finding out, when she was in her 70's, that her mother was no rrrreally her mother. Her mother was a victim of the Spanish flu plague in the early 1900's and she, along with her brother, were put in an orphanage until her father found another wife and mother for his kids.

But my mother learned about that big family secret from her older aunts while on a vacation when they attempted to play a game of family tree. I can only imagine what that "tree" looked like.

So, a curious anomaly, missed by a son who was, maybe, too involved in his own life. She lived until the age of 94 and in spite of that, we still included "Gma Ruth," as she was affectionately known in our universe of friends and family, in as much of our lives as possible. I had three sons, a wife, and a business to attend to, not to mention my own interests. And let's not forget the cat and dog. How much more involved could I be in helping with Mom when my two sisters were nowhere to be found?

Ironically, here I am, in a place so similar to hers. I could be living with a family curse. Do my kids have a lurking, predisposition to this terror? Is it lying in wait for them? Doctors offer no comfort or knowledge to that question. But if I can inherit my parent's looks, why not their illnesses?

Maybe they'll have just the same coincidence as another thirty or so million people with diabetes-induced neuropathy. Welcome to an unwanted club.

I can only hope that my children don't have to experience this curse like my mother and I. But on the other hand, their plight might be lessened and mitigated by the developments of science and technology in the next fifty, or so, years. They shall see, won't they? But nevertheless, it's beyond their control or mine. So, "Hope" is flimsily appropriate. Sorry. I wish them well. Although "hopes and prayers" have been exercised for millennia, we think and expect doctors to perform miracles. But hope, alone, doesn't heal. It's the discoveries of science that enables our realistic expectations.

It also didn't occur to me at the time, but although I may have considered myself the number one concern, there were others experiencing my illness from other perspectives. I, also, wasn't fully tuned into their feelings or needs either. I suppose because every other day was a new issue, test, result, or just a mere unknown; all days were full of fk'g unknowns. It was impossible to catch a breath to think otherwise about something other than myself. Some latest development or result was always occupying my time.

I'm basically a direction kind of guy. I like to have goals and know where I'm going in life. Tell me I've got eight months, or two years to this sentence, and I can prepare. I'll say, "ok, shit happens." But going down a road to the unknown is not really my style. I can't plan for that. Particularly when I'm paying a price, every minute, in pained confinement and difficulty getting around. Who can think right? What's the point of hanging around when considering the cost? Everything has a Return on Investment, and the price to play in this game is getting higher by the day. Maybe I don't want to participate or subject myself to this poorly defined investment.

My sons are, now, perfectly capable of steering their own lives without me, although they may try to make me believe otherwise. But my feelings should be considered too, no? Must I be commanded to devote all of my undying breaths to sharing their existence? Is there a time when someone can turn off the rain and relieve me of my misery? Or am I basically sitting around, waiting for that dying moment, that unavoidable moment? And maybe the beginning of my permanent "holiday."

12

Comedy from Tragedy

Now there's Stop 'n Shop in my life because it's convenient. Nothing's like a visit to the local supermarket. I could browse the aisles endlessly with my fetish for looking at foods, reading ingredients, prices, and just getting ideas. A culinary expedition and certainly convenient for last minute store-needs. Turns out, it is one of many places for my new condition to make things more difficult.

Dee wasn't feeling well one day, and she wanted chicken soup. I decided that I was the man for the job. But THAT was a bad idea. Ya see, they had this old soup display case with three of those pots with covers, the flip-tops with ladles in them... Well, it also had one of those protective plexiglass-like screens (like over salad-bars) in front of the kettles that prevented easy access to ladling out the soup, unless you were a midget to get below the glass!

So, I decided I was going to "reengineer" the thing. I proceeded to lift the glass for easier access, but little did I know, that one side wasn't properly hinged.

Now, for those of you not familiar with the domino effect, that's when one thing basically leads to another and eventually the whole incident then morphs into chaos. When raising the side of the screen that was unhinged, it caused a jerking motion. So, my reflexes kicked in. Not a good reaction in this case because, due to my poor muscular control, I can't stop a reflex. Well, picture this: Me raising and dislodging the glass, the stack of cups went flying, the soup labels ended up in the soup kettles, and I'm left holding the glass. Only, to gently put it down on the next counter...

I was mortified to say the least and figured, as a good honorable citizen with an honest accident, I would a) wish I had a tail to tuck between my legs, and b) tell someone: "spillage in aisle 1." So, I walked, or hobbled, rather, across the store to the service counter and told the manager of the disruption in the soup area caused by some green, big-eyed, monster.

So, they moseyed over and, unphased, proceeded to do the cleanup, totally unmoved by the monster story. Meanwhile, the manager couldn't miss asking if I needed a cover for my soup container. Ha! OK, shit happens. But like they say, lightning strikes twice—right?

Dee's soup, that I worked so hard for, now smartly sitting in the baby seat of my cart, decided that it couldn't hold on when I made an abrupt left turn down an aisle. It went flying out of the cart and across the floor like some *Toy Story* character. That was really too much for my testosterone depleted nerves to handle. This time I just proceeded to the checkout, half a soup container and all. I forgot about the rest of my list. "Cleanup in aisle 6!" Thank you!

As if that weren't enough; as I quickly loaded my car, I forgot to close the trunk until I realized why the interior lights weren't going out. I felt like Woody Allen's Moose on the hood routine. It wakes up in the Lincoln Tunnel after only being grazed by a hunter's bullet. The moose looks at Woody, Woody looks at the moose...

* * *

There are always more funny moments, though. One of the tolls of this affliction is how tired I can get. I believe it's the constant battle of the nerves vs. the muscles or lack thereof. Anyway, I'm sitting in the office chair in the restaurant when I decided to close my eyes and I dozed off. But wouldn't you know, my elbow slips off the arm-rest, which I can't feel, and I fall out of the chair because now I'm so clumsy!

I also find that when I doze or I'm in an early sleep and dreaming, I manipulate my hands as if I'm acting out the dream with the same hand movements. And while closing my eyes to rest peacefully, I can flinch so violently, sometimes poking myself in the face. I feel like a snake with its head cut off and the body still twitching. All weird. Maybe a sleep test is somewhere in the cards. Maybe it's my drug dosage?

With neuropathy, the sensation of feel, touch, and balance are all affected. Consequently, it's necessary to compensate for the missing sense and something else must activate to compensate for the loss.

One vital component becomes the visual, like looking for the horizon to help prevent seasickness. Standing alone, under normal circumstances, one could close their eyes and feel the balance going on in the feet to prevent tipping. Without getting clinical, you'd feel the slight leaning of the body and the leg muscles following the lead of the bottoms of your feet would command a slight adjustment from the leg muscles to stay upright. Of course, this is all dictated by the brain with nerves transmitting signals running the length of the body.

Now, in the dark, I lurch and careen off of walls because I don't have all of my equipment working properly. And when pulling the shirt over my head, if I can't see my way out of the shirt I'll lose my bearings in the darkness, and down I go.

So, I don't have that sense of balance anymore. And it not only affects standing straight up, but it also affects my hands when hold-ing things, like a cup of coffee. Because my hands and wrists are weak, they have a natural tendency to droop. If I'm not looking at the cup, I'm not going to keep that cup of coffee from spilling over. I need to stare at the cup.

Get the picture? Try living like this: that this old dog can learn a new trick?

So, if the wife is pissed at me, she doesn't turn on the night-light over my bedside. In the dark I'm doomed to crash into things. But don't think I don't make enough noise to wake her, finding my way and settling in. Unfortunately, these little body adjustments are taken for granted by most people while I don't even have them. Imagine yourself having to relearn all of these behaviors, just to have some normalcy of life, and that comes with a cost. But now, I need the time and effort to learn this new language.

And for what? So, I can continue the torture? But for how long? 'Till my life runs out because I simply have a built-in expiration time clock like other people? And after all the reconditioning, I die?

C'mon! I'm in a jail-cell. My prison without bars. At various times to family members I brought up the subject of the termination of my life. Bryce, my oldest, had trouble talking to me. He said I was selfish. The rest of the family needed me, he said. But at what cost? To me, I was paying for the privilege to keep going. Both in terms of money and of bodily pain and reliability. Not everyone who wants to do away with their lives suffers from depression. Maybe some of us just can't endure the persistent pain, discomfort, or lack of dignity because you're just falling apart too quickly to keep up? We all deserve a death with dignity. No one should be forced to become a Head-in-the-Bed or feel like a burden.

13

How about a second opinion...

So, after being home from the hospital for about two months, and feeling that my health was only going downhill, my current neuro guy, who was an old multiple sclerosis expert, ran out of steam. He, too, waived his white flag, surrendering to the complexity of the situation, and said go to The Mayo Clinic. I think he was in over his head with his old-school tactics and burdened with a new illness to deal with.

Although he may take credit for suggesting our visit to Mayo, little did he know that we were, proactively, ahead of him. All we needed was his professional referral and it was off to see the Mayo's Wizard of OZ.

This was after, of course, searching for a local neuro guy familiar with my situation. Hey, New York City should have plenty—right? No. And when we were able to make an appointment, it could be months away.

Isn't the big perceived, problem with Canada's "socialized" medicine about the long wait for appointments? Well, maybe because as healthcare becomes available to more people, without expanding the doctor pool, they're simply waiting in line for an appointment! Forget the "label" Socialized. It's a "single-payer" system that has benefits over a "for-profit" system leading to over-aggressive, duplicate practices of expensive, unnecessary, testing procedures. Revenues can either be increased with more procedures or decrease costs with more efficiency while increasing the quantity of patients. Which makes more sense? Treat more people with greater efficiency or less with greater expense? But if you have the "Ben Franklins," as they say, you can buy a battery of tests in one week or less. Probably enough to determine what's ailing you or even me.

With my Dr. "Wormy's" referral, we contacted the Mayo Clinic in Minnesota and were able to get an appointment within two weeks. Mileage points were available, and bodies eager to go. No more: "Squeeze my fingers, raise your arms, touch your nose tricks." So, getting a wish—off we went to The Mayo Clinic in Rochester, MN. I was ready for my "Yellow Brick Road," to see my own *Wizard of Oz*. Or so this Tin Man thought.

We flew out Sunday for a Monday 7a.m. early-morning appointment with an expert in his field and the testing methodically scheduled in advance. It's probably modeled from Federal Express. All patients fly in, processed asap, and sent out when complete. Certainly efficient. But effective?

And why did we arrive on Sunday? Because Rochester, MN is not exactly a popular destination. You take the flight when it's available. And I had to be there before the next morning when the cows were let out of the barn.

The anticipation of the trip was thrilling and overwhelming. Unfortunately, because my immune system was being suppressed with 70mg of Prednisone, I, practically, became the compost for all illnesses and their symptoms. I constantly ran a low fever as a result of a, yet to be detected, chest viral infection and a urinary tract infection. So, I was limp and foggy in a wheelchair when greeting my Wizard. Fortunately, Dee, an NYU trained nurse, was there to be my advocate (and chair pusher). It is really important for a patient not to think they can absorb all the information they're presented with.

It's just not possible, especially when the issue is as complex as mine and your brain has a tendency to get distracted or befuddled.

A sick person needs an advocate—and another pair of ears, with a head in-between, to listen. I was lucky to have both. Monday was also the first day of tests. From blood to electronic needles, to blood pressure tests; they even stripped me down, rubbed me with a brown clay powder, and then baked me at 120F for 40 minutes to see if my sweat turned purple.

Well, that was different. Blueberry muffins couldn't receive better treatment. But it was rather routine testing for a neuropathic patient with Medicare.

Let's just say that Mayo-land in Rochester, MN, is not a cosmopolitan city. The corn grows up to the runway and the City Center is a short car ride down the road. I almost expected to see *Scarecrow* on the way. The town seems to exist for the Mayo Clinic and its related facilities.

Now don't get me wrong, although the renowned Mayo Clinic may be located in Bum FK, USA, the Mayo Clinic may also be the top facility in the country; hands down, or so we imagined.

The Clinic reeks of money, equipment, facilities, knowledge. Their reputation (good marketing?) precedes them. The military discipline of their procedures, testing, and patient handling are unparalleled. They move armies, I mean armies of people from blood tests through all the same testing regimes I experienced in NY, plus some. There must have been 100 chairs in the waiting areas for most tests, and at least 400 or so chairs with people in them, and multiple nurses in the blood testing area. It was like a well-run Costco of hospitals. Everyone moving in some musically, choreographed, Rockettes-type, lockstep. It was like a 50's/60's *Mad Men* office landscape. All visiting patients showed up with charts, processed, and, pirouetting left, consulted with their doctors. Not to say some patients may have been disappointed with the results or something else. We were certainly impressed. They even had a pianist and, at times, a singer in the lobby!

But it occurred to me that this must have been one of the secret formulas for healthcare to make money: Think about the revenues produced from all of those vials of blood; each one like those built-in shopping, on-line fees. They add up fast.

Whereas in the NYC hospital they performed, what seemed like, a disorganized battery of tests; At Mayo they performed a more so-phisticated battery focused, with the latest equipment, on my neu-rological condition. In all fairness, though, Saini was starting from discombobulated scratch, with the liver and all. The Mayo Clinic had a head start with Saini's preliminary work, and their toys were the best. But if Mt. Saini was a facility equipped to handle neuro-pathic patients, where was the specialized equipment; like a "Tilt Table?" Theirs seemed like some portable Black 'n Decker power tool.

Unfortunately, we were not aware of what was missing; probably like most people when being admitted to a hospital on an emergency basis. I'll bet few emergency room patients don't or can't ask: "First, can I see your facilities?" And, if they do, they're NOT referring to the bathroom!

* * *

When we met with the Doctor, he gave us good news and some no-news. The good news was that apparently the LGi1 antibody cells were wiped out of my body by at least one of the medications ad-ministered during my Mt. Saini stay. They believe it may have been the Rituximab. The no-news was that no one can say as to when this sentence in my cell will end.

But as testing results came in, a clearer picture emerged for us: We would be going home with the task of finding local doctors to administer a Mayo driven plan for treatment. As we entered the plane and were sitting in our seats, comforted that we came, Dee's phone rang and rang. Should we or shouldn't we answer? "Oh, what the heck, answer it."

14

"What? You want us to do what? Where? When? Sure."

It was my doctor and he wanted us to deplane and immediately go to the St. Mary's/Mayo hospital emergency room. At that point I wanted to cry—but couldn't, not to mention that when recollecting the moment, it still makes my eyes tear. Apparently, an infection showed up in my blood that could be toxic. Imagine how that story appeared to the airlines, particularly the luggage vis a vis the terrorism aspect. Fortunately, the airline was understanding, until it came to the ticket—penalties?

But at that moment, I really did want to cry. Still, apparently not in touch with my unjustified feelings at the time. I suppose, I was probably still in denial because no one would tell me the truth, or let's say, what's most likely in store to occur in my future so I can process it. Like, after almost six months, c'mon, enough was enough!

With this infection I was at risk for going septic. A 500 Fungi reading of some sort on somebody's meter. Biopsy, cat scan, what now was to be ordered? "But I just had that!" Too many chefs in the kitchen? And the surprise? After admission to the emergency room, and an IV stuck in my elbow so it couldn't bend, up to room 506 in the Mayo hospital—a private room with a view. Sound familiar?

More tests scheduled to see the extent of the mass found in my lung. Can you imagine? Suppose the call came after we took off? Go back to Hackensack, NJ, and start telling my story to *their* emergency room? A fourth facility, and how many more unfamiliar-with-my-case doctors to get up to speed?

Was the Dec. 2017 cough the onset of my illness? Could all of this have been avoided with a more diligent treatment in the first place a year ago—maybe with a more comprehensive and accessible patient database that followed a protocol? A database that could have alerted the docs to a possible overdose of medication and results from already completed tests? Could the hundreds-of-thousands of dollars in expenses that all of you taxpayers paid through Medicare also have been avoided by keeping track of all of a patient's information with a database? This database could eliminate the unnecessary and overlapping expenses of retesting to constantly starting from "go" all the time for that "second opinion?"

Overnight led to five more days of incarceration, confusion, testing, another biopsy. All for CYA?

On top of that, adding insult to injury, the new staff at Mayo hospital prescribed a medication that would cost $3,500 a month to clear up my infection. But Medicare wouldn't cover the expense.

The cost of time and stress was, now, becoming the price for living. But after some doctor's reconsideration of the prescription, and not confident that this drug would "do it," they said it really wasn't necessary.

Really, again? Imagine the fickleness of thought and how this must drive people nuts. Not to mention, some people would be tortured by the unobtainable expense of this medication. But the medical industry is counting on people never batting an eye, because of "Doctor's recommendations," about taking this unnecessary and expensive medicine. Who has the "balls" to refuse a doctor's recommendation?

I was at wits end and I wanted to go home. I was pushing for a release date but yielding to common sense when necessary. I am uncomfortable, not insane.

It was more than my own discomfort that made me need to leave. I really felt for the wife, alone in some local motel while I'm back in a St. Mary's hospital. It *was* time to leave. The party was getting stale and tired. Dee was now spending the nights alone in some spooked out motel 1,200 miles away from home with me in another hospital with only the sounds of the corn rustling in the breeze at night. I think if the shoes were on different feet, I would even feel just as creeped out with the prospect: "Here I am, all alone in a cornfield." Jason of *Friday the 13th* couldn't be far away.

We returned home the next Thursday. Another week lost to the unknown. I saw that rerun already and I was succumbing to the runaround.

We landed at the grimy, congested Newark airport, just the same as coming home from Florida or practically anywhere else. It was still the gateway to home. Rochester, MN wouldn't cut it.

But we were armed with some good news, some optimism, and a goal to finally hit the ground running. But that plan means IVIG once a week in NYC. And I'm the eternal optimist, the pragmatist's definition of "hope." Get adjusted to being home, no more ice cream two times a day, a flight of stairs to traverse, and a restaurant to run. What could be more fun?

15

Home with the "Homies."

I'm an engineer by training and a builder by profession. My problem-solving abilities follow the same medical solving organization of ideas—just a different language. A diagnosis seems to follow like any other discipline of going through a series of logical gates or paths leading to a conclusion.

I was being patient, sometimes stoic, sometimes noncommittal because no one has a definitive answer. And I didn't want to be some conspiracy theorist based on some inconclusive evidence. No cause or connection to a series of events that can explain my illness, along with everyone's changed life. Therefore, there seems to be no course of action to recovery; because the doctors need a diagnosis first, regardless that the symptoms may closely mimic similar illnesses.

So, I'm in limbo. Now, almost nine months later after entering the hospital, the symptoms seem to be getting worse. No commitment to recovery. Forget finding a cure. At this point I merely want comfort of mind to know where I'm going. It's all getting more hopeless. I just can't seem to wrap my arms around this illness to get some closure or course of attack. The doctors won't commit either because they don't know WTF I have, and are fearful of not covering their asses if they give false or misleading info. They remain evasively mute or non-committal. Talk about confidence-building.

Although sometimes we step in shit—get hit by a car, yada yada, some of us can clean up—others less so. What kind of shit did I step into? The neuropathic jail-cell seems to, incrementally, tighten daily. But the doctors either minimize my concerns or are incapable of taking action. Without a diagnosis, I guess they're impotent like me!

* * *

The next challenge was to find local doctors to take up the treatment and guidance in NJ. No small feat.

With the rarity of my circumstance, it was, and is, difficult to find at least knowledgeable players. One internist said, "Ok, I'll take you on, but I'm changing my practice's business model to include a $1,500 additional fee per year to make sure you get the attention you'll need." I said, "Bye!"

I realized, that's what patient care has come to for the less fortunate and those not on Medicare. The "money" gets the attention. The rest? Welcome to Tony Soprano's NJ medical option.

If I don't have a definitive diagnosis as to recovery, then I can't pull any plugs on myself. But I need a carrot on a stick to keep me going. My drive will run out unless I can find purpose in the store, sharing my health experience, or maybe something currently unknown. My memories are all that motivate me. There's little that I would consider new and exciting. I need something constructive to continue existing—not to live in unproductive misery at the expense of myself and others.

It is a simple plus-or-minus situation. Imagine your feet being wrapped in balls of cotton with duct tape around and then shoved into shoes with balled socks. That's part of my current "fun." It's like walking on stumps. Add to that, compression stockings made from itchy wool wrapped around your hands and forearms to the armpits. And then, put on a suit made of tight-fitting vest material where every move reminds you that you are inside a turtle's shell, some medieval metal body armor, or constrained in Mummy's cloth. Now, attach a stiff neck, add on being tired most of the time, and you're in my skin. Aaand the answer is?

It's tough to keep up the fight. I don't have the energy or even the ability. Much of my time now revolves around my medical needs. No time to spare for a restaurant business that requires an exhausting amount of attention and imagination, even by the standards of a younger person! I lose my train of thought.

Meanwhile the doctor-visits and bills keep coming. It's gotta be close to the million-dollar mark. Without Medicare and secondary BCBS we would be doomed for bankruptcy. Just put all expenses on the Medicare credit card and never look at a bill! What a relief not to be concerned. So *what* if I can't pay a bill, or I'm forced into bankruptcy? Why should I be any more concerned than those corporate titans declaring bankruptcy, multiple times even, and then restarting under a another business? But imagine foregoing a meal or two, maybe more, in lieu of having to pay for needed medicine. And is that the world we want to live in? How can we ignore such compounded misery?

Fortunately, before entering the hospital with this avalanche of an illness, serendipitously, I also arranged for a small-business loan for the business.

Money or business was probably the last thing on anyone's mind. But as the confusion mounted, the bills kept coming...

So, although I had other plans for the loan, it ended up being used as an emergency fund to pay *all* bills; thinking it'll all get sorted out later by the accountant.

One's health is a human right. It becomes a Catch-22 pitting work to pay the bills against staying healthy to work; while the fortunate enough few can't even count all the zeros on their bank statements, regardless of their illnesses. Many bought some gas from you, a computer, phone, a car? Give some back! Money gluttons and hoarders are less than fashionable nowadays. Do we want to say that the best of days as a society are behind us? Or do the niggard money hoarders and gluttons eventually feel some compassion that they have enough at the expense of the less fortunate; regardless of their feelings of entitlement. Shame on them.

Rainy days sometimes come with little warning, especially the long and painful rainy years. And I also understand that too many cannot even establish a "rainy day fund." And that sucks, too. But if we had a universal healthcare, maybe most wouldn't find themselves tortured as to how these bills get paid. So, it is a foregone conclusion that too many will be playing the unnecessary Russian Roulette wheel with healthcare. And the mere retort that unbridled capitalism is the answer, needs to be reexamined for obsolescence of thought. People are more than dollars and cents or the unyielding "American Dream" of profit or fail. WE are all certainly not afforded the same opportunity to achieve the basics of human existence. If those at the top of government can make policy that affects people and their jobs, our politicians can manipulate and screw up all they want as long as the public's basic health and security survives.

* * *

I try to find the humor and laugh at myself. One day it was the chicken soup, another the coffee cup spills over, or the wine glass perilously droops and spills on the floor. Today the blueberries went all over the place because my hands jerk. What a mess. What a dichotomous laugh that followed; and what it all masks. I laugh at myself because the blueberries, the chicken soup, the coffee cups, and the wine glasses, and all the other smorgasbord of slips are all self-deprecating dopy moments, funny slap-stick incidences—something I laughed at while growing up and watching the likes of Abbot and Costello, The Three Stooges, or Lucille Ball. Now, I'm in the movie. They are genuine funnies when it's out of your control. But beneath the surface lurks the deeper troubling voice. What's causing the pain? What's causing the family duress? What's the root of the suicide wish? And is there an answer here? A day doesn't pass that I wouldn't yell an expletive out of frustration or get pissed off with my newfound, unannounced, crippling condition.

Each of my three boys exhibited something different when it came to addressing and dealing with my illness. Each loving and concerned, but I guess I couldn't tune into their needs or issues as much as I suppose I superficially tried, if at all. Bryce brought food treats for me along with a positive spin on my condition. "Chocolate Brittles" were a real hit because of the Prednisone induced craving for sweets.

Jesse, as loving as always, the soon-to-be oral surgeon, was very interested in the medical aspect although somewhat hamstrung because he was more in Boston than New York. And Landon, couldn't be more willing to help and set me up with technical support as well as his additional loving attention. I don't think there is a luckier father with these three guys.

Yet I know from my own experience with my father and his early cancer days in the hospital: It's weird seeing your "invincible" dad in a vulnerable state of health. If the reality check doesn't click in then, it eventually will.

I'm sorry my simple humanity, confronted by vulnerabilities I was unprepared for, prevented their feelings from hardly entering my mind. I suppose it follows that when one has frost bite, the blood goes to the core first, the limbs last, no matter how important those limbs are.

At times like these, friendships change, even lifelong ones. Besides, how close can friends be if they don't call you in over a year to see how you're doing? Pretending to be insulted is no excuse. What can be more important between friends than being there for a time like this? Are they cowards because they don't know how to deal with the uncomfortable illness of a long-time "friend," or is this some unrelated character trait on their part that results in dismissing "old friends?" I'll just have to update my own programming and move on.

But Dee and the family is a whole other conversation. Not only am I grappling with a life-changing affliction, but the family is also dealing with it and their mostly secret thoughts about it.

Dee has been my sidekick. If I were alone on an island and allowed any three things, I would pick Dee for the first—and forget the other two. I wake up every day, blessed, to be with her for another 24 hours. I understand what a love she is to me. A little "heavy" with shtick, perhaps, but I can hardly imagine what goes through her mind other than what we've dared to speak about.

Do I ask? I'm all consumed with the illness and its related topics: like what's the status of the physical changes; the tests; the doctors, the medications and their side effects; the mental disposition being afflicted; now add a complete layer of "the store," and ALL of its related issues; and then of all things, the thought about my possibly ending this nightmare—suicide. Maybe one would think it's a little too much? Yes, the infirmed can become selfish and occupied, but surely not without provocation .

Ask Dee what she thinks about my health: how it affects our lives together, not to mention hers; how it has changed the mobility for us as a couple; what care I do or will need; the loss of our sex lives; the simple touching that communicates so much more.

It's all pretty confusing and fucked up to say the least. Is "challenging" an understatement? It's more of a tornado in the brain. Funny, I never got a headszup in school as to the shit all will experience.

This ailment made me realize the act of the touch goes deeper than just the surface. It's something I think we take for granted as with probably most other things—until they're taken away. I've always been told that I have "good hands," whether caressing one's toes, feet, whatever, or beyond. Finding the pressure-points and slowly massaging gives a unique connection between a couple. I always enjoyed and received as much, if not more, gratification from giving the pleasure as the one receiving it. It was the connection between the two of us that was the gift that kept giving—and now it's gone.

Apparently executive functioning in the brain is also affected by this neurological affliction. Not only do I become befuddled with the simplest of chores, like sorting papers into categories, because I've lost that "neurological glue." I sometimes get confused with the organization of thoughts, if I don't forget the idea in the first place. It's like one thought gets pushed aside by another, to be misplaced or forgotten, like passing through one ear and out the other—transient (for now, it generally comes back if I retrace my mental steps, or so I imagine). The brain is an amazing organ. But are my problems affected by illness, medication, or just age-related?

I'm still driving my car with slight adjustments. Weeeee. Although I have trouble feeling the wheel. I can grip it, so it doesn't fly out of my hands, which it's done. Occasionally, my foot slips off of the gas or brake pedal. I find I have to reset its position because I've noticed I sometimes step on the brake instead of the gas. At other times, while the car is in park, I belatedly hear the engine roar because I inadvertently step on the gas. But I've also learned to compensate for lack of feel for the pedals using the visual. I can see how fast I'm stopping or how fast I'm traveling by observing the speedometer as well as the relative speed to my surroundings. I still feel safe for myself and others. Otherwise, I don't think I would be stubborn enough to continue driving.

I believe my mother felt compelled to give up her license after having a car accident and nearly running over someone. She hated giving up some control over her life. It meant that she wouldn't be able to drive and visit the kids; not to mention that she would be beholden to others for transportation. Further, as a widow, it was a realization to her that not being able to drive meant more time at home—alone. It may take an accident, an earthquake, or near enough close call to change my mind about driving. But I don't think I would be a strenuous protester. It would be a rationale for less responsibility. Sort of "easing" into a new life with less stress...

Even though Dee and the boys, apparently, don't mind taking over the driving. I think they do it because maybe they don't trust me and driving makes them feel better. But I'm ok with that. I won't tell.

How do I feel? Not angry. Only frustration at what I'm incapable of doing. No one did this to me so how can I really feel anger toward anyone? Maybe angry at the internist who continued the Augmentin in spite of some red flags in the medical community regarding its repeated use, and for ignoring the reported tingly sensation that didn't get recognition and timely treatment. The neurologist at Mt. Saini who thought he had a handle on my condition just because he was a neurologist, but was too old to realize otherwise; and maybe my Neurologist at Mayo because he celebrated the elimination of my LGi1, without doing a follow-up for another possible culprit; or maybe my first pulmonologist because he, I'm sure, hardly thought to do a chest x-ray or cat scan which most likely would have shown the lung growth. But the path to achieving satisfaction on that "angry" front is not a quick fix. I am angry. Why me? M-fkrs! But it's like screaming at some unknown character on a Yahoo message board! What's the point?!

From the NY Times review of:

THE UNWINDING OF THE MIRACLE.....by Julie Yip-Williams

> "We might be tempted to assume that these books were written mostly for the writers themselves, as a way to make sense of a frightening diagnosis and uncertain future; or for their families, as a legacy of sorts, in order to be known more fully while alive and kept in mind once they were gone.
>
> By dint of being published, though, they were also written for us — strangers looking in from the outside. From our seemingly safe vantage point, we're granted the privilege of witnessing a life-altering experience while knowing that we have the luxury of time. We can set the book down and mindlessly scroll through Twitter, defer our dreams for another year or worry about repairing a rift later, because our paths are different.
>
> Except that's not entirely true. Life has a 100 percent mortality rate; each of us will die, and most of us have no idea when. Therefore, Yip-Williams tells us, she has set out to write an "exhortation" to us in our complacency: Live while you're living, friends."

* * *

One needs a sense of purpose to exist. I had my building business, my book, restaurant, rowing for exercise, and recipes. Plenty to do and feel proud and purposeful. The mind was occupied and not dwelling on the "Woe is me." I raised three boys into men. I know the pressure now of the role model. How do I think about terminating my life? It certainly wouldn't be an expression of giving up without cause or justification. There wouldn't be a reason to hate me. I'm in a jail without a crime. How about Habeas Corpus? What means of escape are there, except facing the indeterminable sentence of time? Every contract has a termination date. I don't get even that except by default. Hate me for what?

I still need a purpose. Whether it's dreaming of recipes or managing a business, writing a book. Unless the pain is unbearable, find a purpose. Sitting in a chair and just "hoping" isn't going to change anything...

Without a brain, what would my future be like? For those truly afflicted, I understand the dreaded imprisonment. It's a measure of our compassion and who we are as people to help the young live their lives and grow. We need to give them the space and resources to become something. But what of those who have lived a life, like me? I'm ok to move on. The Kanyes and Kardashians will come and go. Make space, funds, and resources for the living.

And don't forget to read: "Living Long by Diane Perish."

Forget those promises you made to yourself about traveling or living a certain life when retiring.

Forget it, because, like me, getting hit broadside with my condition dashed all expectations going forward. We're many times derailed in our dreams and goals. So, this is not a journal about dying. I'm one of the last ones to give up. Do all and whenever you can, lest you may wind up disappointed and with the druthers later on. I just can't and I don't know when to "sell" for being the eternal optimist.

It's almost, do I hang up five minutes before someone picks up with a cure? Or let's be real, the cavalry ain't comin' to me anymore, and they all went home long ago.

We could write about making every minute of life count to the fullest or for that matter, once you're dead, for those who have not contributed, does it really matter? It was obviously a personal choice how to use one's time.

From the same article about Julie Yip-Williams:

> " "I didn't deserve this! My children didn't deserve this!" She frets about the "Slutty Second Wife" her husband will one day marry and the pain her daughters will experience in her absence. And, near the end, she oscillates between being game to try every possible treatment and accepting that nothing will keep her alive. "

As a practical matter, the world will go on, with or without us all, at some point, even if we're kicking and screaming on the way. Think the herds of animals with their predators and illnesses. Shit does happen. But how do we want to be remembered and how did we address the end game?

* * *

On our February, family vacation in St. Martin, I'm in someone's $1mil condo, with no phones or internet, looking for a different place, and not wanting to be trapped next to an airport. Besides, there are no elevators or handrails present, to say the least. Obviously, building codes for safety measures are not as stringent as good ole' USA. A few steps from the beach? A few steps in my condition is an unassisted marathon or another mountain to climb. Is that what

I want to do on a vacation in my condition? Thanks, sensible and in-clusive people for the contributions to the betterment of all people with the ADA (American Disability Act). Why should we live in a world excluding less-advantaged people? That's compassion.

Most of my life on vacation I would zip around, unfettered, walking endlessly to wherever time and circumstances allowed. Now, I'm at the mercy of others. At some point I understand I have to give up control when it comes to planning. Most liked our planned trips, and I didn't know otherwise. But it's difficult to abruptly cede a po-sition when one has been doing it for years without any major issues. For now, the best I can hope for is to be included in the ride.

But you know there's always some humor as usual, if you can find it. We're sitting in a beautiful waterfront setting, and as we're all talking, my finger gets stuck in the coffee-cup handle. So, there I am, trying to listen to the conversation, and I'm rattling the cup trying to remove my finger. Two seagulls look at each other...

16

Back to business

Day 270—And I finally went to the ophthalmologist and found out I need cataract operations. Just keep piling it on.

Cataract surgery comes in twos because I have two eyes and who does only one? It's just not that simple. First, one has to be fitted for the lenses. That, I'm told, takes a 2-3-hour doctor's office exam to measure for the lenses. Then, the procedure, which takes a half an hour can only be done one at a time, with eye patches and all. Then, the second eye can be done with some follow-up, of course. Creepy. But the ingenuity of the human brain certainly shines with the advanced technological display of medical equipment.

Cutting the eye to insert a lens sounds like the opening razor-blade scene in Luis Bunuel's *An Andalusian Dog*. Catch it on YouTube, and, trust me, it may give you second thoughts.

The eye exam revealed that my cataracts were apparently not an emergency. Always nice to have one medical issue not be a crisis. Although I would have an operation to remove the clouded lens, I would still need glasses for reading. So, the doctor said I can try new ones after getting the eyelids surgically raised. Now, THAT'S on the to-do list.

But guess who has to take me and pick me up? Of course, the wife. I hate being dependent on her and it's a source of friction. How would you like your day to be controlled by someone else? I get it, every once in a while, but this is becoming too frequent. With my condition I half-heartedly joke again: "Now, how much ya love me?"

Meanwhile, catering orders to the city for the store are picking up. GREAT news! More revenue. Just more logistics and execution to think about. That gives me some sense of purpose to fight on.

By all rights, I should be looking for a new location for the store, closer to the city, but one that I can also take advantage of the demographics. It would be nice to have tables and a chance to increase local catering. A liquor license would seal the deal, but NJ just doesn't get it yet. Liquor licenses are also difficult to obtain.

I believe being in New York City would be a homerun, but I can't imagine paying the crazy-high rent and risking it. Remember, I'm not doing this with an IPO or plenty of seed capital and money to burn as per the latest business model—raise enough money, to buy market share on the hype, to pay years of losses. Smoked is all homegrown, organic, small business survival. Nearby there is a local town with high-rises, a major hospital, and a county courthouse. THAT'S a population of 50,000 AND a potential daily rotation of new customers! All the while about 20 minutes closer to the city for deliveries. Sounds like the right move to me.

There's also something about the excitement of a new venture. Figuring out the weak points of an existing one and improving on it all creates a gravitational pull for me.

But now I have to think about getting out of the existing lease, negotiating a new one in a different location, outfitting a new space, and everything costing new money. Not what I'd really like to be doing now at my age and health status. I'd like to be on a beach with a Pina Colada and little to think about except my own "72 dancing virgins;" (or even "raisins," as believed to have been misinterpreted). But that's not realistic. At this point a mini-parasol would do.

* * *

I had the occupational therapist test the sensation in my fingers because I've suspected that the usefulness of my hands has diminished. The doctors have told me to ignore my "feelings," as if things can get worse before getting better.

The results were not encouraging. As she claimed she was testing each finger, I believed she wasn't moving. I said that I always felt the same sensation in the same finger regardless that she WAS roving her instrument from finger to finger. NOT GOOD! I couldn't feel properly in the other fingers, and I couldn't manipulate them with efficiency. They were becoming a jumble of signals and therefore useless.

I, also, thought getting rid of the antibody was a good thing since there wouldn't be the reason for my nerves to continue to suffer. The nerve degeneration would cease, and it would just be a matter of time before regeneration occurs to restoration. Or, so I thought. Must be wishful thinking on my part—huh? Because what do I know, I'm just the patient and I'm supposed to disregard my feelings. I didn't think this was good, either. So, I got a refill of my amitriptyline (an antidepressant and sleeping pill)—just in case.

Now it's time to write the monthly checks for the store bills. Only I can't write. So, I do the best I can to annotate the amounts on the envelopes and Dee can do what I used to: write the checks or enter them for online payment. More theft of her time. Another reason for her to resent my illness. "Now how much ya love me?" I'd rather be doing the orders for next week and thinking about new recipes, but I'm slowed down with this affliction.

And Dee is dragged along for the ride. I just don't have the energy or the time to do it all. The drive yes, but not the energy. Grrrr. And Dee? Don't ask what lurks beneath her surface beyond the usual checkbook fears. But, regardless of all the "noise," I know we're in love.

* * *

Day 286—I'm really feeling miserable. Medieval, body-suit torture 'n all. I go to physical therapy and I'm convinced it's not for growth or repair. Merely maintenance. My hands can't even hold chopsticks. That was my dexterity barometer. They feel stiff and numb; the sticks just roll out of my hands. You can't tell me I'm getting better.

I'm also convinced that with the lack of urgency with my case, we're all waiting around for the earth to move, like nerve regeneration. Until that time we all go through the motions of tests to see the progress in either direction for where this thing is heading. Why bother? Just give me an eye-mask, earphones, valium, and another MRI just to keep up the momentum. Let's make the effort to appear to solve this illness.

* * *

My Mayo doctor recommended I get an autonomic reflex screen to be included in the latest assessment of my condition. Sounds reasonable enough—find a local doctor or institution to administer the test—and report it all to the interested parties.

Noooo. Apparently, there are no facilities in Northern NJ to administer this test. Unfortunately, my local neurologist doesn't have the equipment, and the major hospitals in Bergen county don't either. Imagine, in the, supposedly, "richest county of the United States," these "major" health facilities don't, not even one, have the ability to administer this test. Huh?

After exhausting the possibilities of local institutions for the test, I called for an autonomic reflex screen to another major hospital facility, and did the lady lie to me!? She told me that their machine was broken and didn't even know if it would be repaired in two months! Ok, plausible, but who knows in today's environment. You're a major facility and they don't know when a critical piece of machinery needed for the practice of their trade will be restored to usefulness? How about, make sure it's repaired within days! Or did they tell me it was out of order because they couldn't accommodate extra patients soon enough? That's not honest!

But wait, she was equipped to immediately provide the names and phone numbers of three local hospitals in NYC. All I had to do was call one.

So, I did; the facility where I originally spent three months. I also emailed my ex-doctor from that hospital to see if he could arrange for the test as my original co-physician. I called, left a message, and no return call. I thought he was concerned. Maybe more like a jilted lover? I guess they wrote me off once again. Or for that matter, maybe they didn't even have the equipment!

Fortunately, I located another institution in NYC who could do the test. But they can only give an appointment three plus months out! This whole Neuro specialty seems to be at a snail's pace—NO urgency to go nowhere. I mean, if wrinkled skin is a given as a sign of aging, why is organ, or systems failure over time, any different? Aren't aging and systems-breakdown a part of life? They're maybe dodgeable, but not unavoidable.

Doesn't say much for the prognosis of my condition, does it? If I'm a really lost cause, along with others like me, what's the point in the investment of the equipment if there's no positive feedback or constructive results to learn from the tests? So, where are we going with this? What do we hope to achieve with this "Frankenstein-like" obsession to extend life and improve living conditions for the some? Eternal life for people with an overabundance of money, and misery for the less fortunate? Who are really the deciders here? Where's the E Pluribus Unum? "Out of many, one."

A little cynical? Perhaps, but totally possible..

I would say profit to the facility is the motivating factor. I'm getting a queasy feeling about profit motivated healthcare. I get that capitalism drives a weeding out process for successful or unsuccessful businesses. But to apply the same "survival of the fittest" standards to who gets to survive and who doesn't seems a little cold, don't ya think? Healthcare is like a utility—everyone needs it. Imagine if the power company wasn't regulated and, like a monopoly, they could raise prices at will, so only the well-off would benefit?

* * *

I miss the ability to feel Dee, to caress. The envelopes and papers can wait. Yes, I can go through the motions; but there's no backup feeling to me. The connection is lost. But not by choice. I feel if I attempted to caress her it would be like using sandpaper to rub a baby's butt. I'm just not into sex using a silicone potholder. Wrong guy!

Day 288-Saw the neuro guy today for the EMG and follow-up results on the last MRI. Now, I walk "like a drunken sailor," so he says. As if he "gets it." I walk more like Vincent D'Onofrio's "Edgar the Bug" from *Men in Black*. So, good news and bad again. It's not in the brain. Bad news: he sees some inflammation in the spine and needs a new MRI of the whole spine. Back to the MRI. Back to laying rigid when the machine clanks around me. Amy Winehouse's, "Going back to rehab—no, no, no!" Yes, yes, yes. Valium day, earplugs, panic button, music, and eye-patch, again, for sure.

So, if I have been complaining of my condition getting worse, why didn't someone do the test earlier? And if the spine shows inflammation, what's next, another spinal tap to show what's creating the inflammation? If it doesn't show in the blood, like the LGi1, it shows in the spinal fluid, right? There's no smile on my face, right now. How does all of this illness stuff get sorted out and solved? I feel like I'm caught spinning in a washing machine.

And because of the recurrence or advancement of the neuropathy, I felt weaker and uninterested in PT or OT. So, we've decided to cut back therapy to once a week because Medicare will only cover up to a max of about $3,000 per annum and we believe we're at about $2,000 already. Best to save some firepower, so we all agree. Besides, my blood-pressure was about 92/62 at therapy. Not exactly a reading conducive to exercise.

As a matter of fact, after I left, I pulled the car into a parking lot about 3 minutes from home and snoozed for half an hour. I just couldn't make it all the way without dozing off and risking an accident. Not good. Not even organizing this week's store orders or working on this narrative was interesting... Today, I clearly gave up. Where's my "purpose?"

The hands are worse and pathetic. It's difficult to even deal with toilet paper, if you know what I mean. Really gross! But what's the choice? We learn to cope. Now, I have to solve a major problem that ordinarily wouldn't be given a second thought. What's the point of relearning everything—and then I die? What do I gain for the cost of my humiliation and the loss of dignity? A cookie with the grandkids? Ah! They're just loveable little brats anyway! But "Baba Bob" can certainly be proud of his kids, and theirs, from wherever he is.

Day 291—worked my ass off in the store today—12 hours. I'm obsessed with making *SMOKED* into a successful catering business. We had our orders from last week and on top of that got two orders for the city today. We're order junkies, so we just had to take them all. Hey—mo' money. But as busy as we were today with the two orders, they really stretched us for time—and we blew it. We took on too much. But because it was a small order, I didn't mind the penalty rather than decline an order while seeking customer recognition.

Meanwhile, since Columbia Presbyterian's machine is broken, I'm now recommended to get a test at NYU. But wait, the doctor calls back, yet can't see me until June. I hung up, pissed, after saying I could be dead by then. Many think we have a better healthcare system than Canada. Who's spinning the tale?

So, after calling my doctor's secretary, she said just make the appointment and they'll call to get a better date. I hate having to be my own secretary in my condition. But I had to tuck my tail between my legs and call back. I had to explain and tell her about my rare affliction. "Oh my!" she said, with hardly a Broadway-worthy response.

WTF—nobody cares—it's not about me—right? I'm just a peripheral or secondary concern—just a body part of their job. But I was not in any state of mind to be jumping through hoops.

Day 299 or about 430,560 minutes. But like they say, who's counting? Yes, apparently, I am, but now mostly out of boredom. I'm tired. I have my urinary infection back again being that I'm immunocompromised; and the autonomic component of the illness also affects the bladder. Maybe it's all a lost cause. All I can think about are my two doctors looking at each other, like a couple of dazed seagulls...

Day 301 had a couple of surprises. First, going to my physical therapy and occupational therapy, I find out that in a couple of visits my PT runs out with Medicare. OT has already run down the clock for reimbursements. The therapists miscalculated. That vapid phrase: "Oops! So sorry." That means, realistically, I can either pay for my own therapy on a private basis or do nothing. Apparently, despite the improvements in my physical rehab, I am still a long way from my pre-illness condition by a longshot. So, I am confronted with paying out of pocket the rest of the year, until Medicare starts again next year, and for what? Or I can injure myself, most likely by falling, and end up reentering the hospital, only to restart the whole process all over again. Since all seems futile, maybe I'll just take the passive-aggressive approach, take back my dignity, and decline their goose chase.

Something is wrong with the system. Better to have maintenance and preventative care than spend more for necessary treatment—right? Well, that's not been the case here.

* * *

On March 30, Dee threw an intimate Saturday-night birthday party for me. It was one with about a dozen people who comprised the core of my past year's closest friends. We toasted them as the core of love and friendship; with Dee the heart of the body. She just made the worst that much better. The boys were beyond great—preparing a Spanish themed meal—cooking all day. Perhaps they may have bit off more than they expected but it was another Bob event of which all participated with much love. My family just blows me away. I'm very fortunate for their love and attention, in spite of how, sometimes, short tempered and nasty I can be.

Never did I expect that going into my 70th would I come out in this shape. I'm not sure where I'm headed or where this leads us all. The mission is to complete the journey wherever it takes us, sort of like the video games the kids play today. Crazy stuff keeps coming and we all have to learn to traverse the onslaught of challenges while life and its surprises continue. The tests, the control ceded to doctors and third parties, the termination of funds and programs; all to be turned into a daily flatulence. Pass "Go" each morning, roll the dice, and let one rip.

* * *

We have four nice-sized catering orders to get out this week for delivery to the city. I'm pleasantly preoccupied. If this continues, I dream more that the smart move would be to relocate closer to the city and have a location large enough to have more tables. Now, how do we find such a place and value the extra space required along with the associated costs? But I act like I'm a forty-year-old in my prime—not someone who just turned seventy and has health issues to boot! My conundrum is terribly frustrating. But there are plenty of entrepreneurs older than I that still pursue the excitement of the challenge. Making money can be fun and preoccupying, for sure. But the question is, where do I get the funds for this potential move? Where do I get the human resources? And where do I get the energy, among other necessities, to execute this plan? On top of that, now, I have to reread: *Deep in Debt, by Owen A. Lott.* This illness compels me to confront some unexpected, crossroad of life. It was a totally random knuckleball.

* * *

So, I get a call today from my local neuro guy's secretary that he had a Friday night phone conversation with my Mayo guy, and wanted to set up a half-hour meeting tomorrow. Unfortunately, I have a delivery tomorrow for the store that conflicts and the wife needs off and suggested doing the doctor appointment another time. Easier said than done. But to keep sanity among the weary, I cancelled the meeting and took my chances on rescheduling the doctor. Dee is at wits end and today was no better. I'm going to be in this condition regardless of what's done on an immediate basis. The recognition of an illness creates a compulsive response, even though any effort might be futile. So, what's the rush to see a doctor? Her sanity is obviously far more important at this point. But there comes a time when staying at the party too long starts to outweigh the benefits of going out a winner.

Do I want my legacy to be about the misery surrounding the end of my life, or the memories remain of a good Dad? How do I want to be remembered? How can I be reliable and dependable if I can't remember, or I make those innocent errors? "The evil lives long after…"

I know the future of your memories. You can remember me as a virile dad, or as a weak, confused, passed-over, old man, wasting away. My preference, I went out on top. The BBQ is over, and we went home; not stayed around until the tables were cleared and the garbage was thrown out.

In the meantime, the hands still aren't learning how to cooperate. Personal hygiene suffers the most. From toothpaste dribbling to shmearing while brushing; to aiming and snaring my food on a shaking fork, and anything else requiring hand dexterity that can ignore my neuromuscular discoordination. If it all came down to only a little extra toothpaste on the brush because of the shaking hands, there would be little to talk about.

The other day, coming back from shopping, I tried to be helpful and help unload the truck. When will I learn that I seem to be making more work for my staff when they have to clean up after me? This time it was the jar of olives. RIGHT out of my hands, they flew like some invisible menace just yanked them away. Onto the floor, sans cap, liquid, and half the olive-jar—pimentos 'n all! So, I sheepishly picked up the now half-filled jar of olives and offered them to Erik. I felt badly, for him, more for his well-being than mine. What does he need me for?

In my letter to Mayo a couple of months ago, I asked if the Doc thought it was prudent to biopsy the lung to see the material that was there if there's any relationship to the antibody or what attacked my Myelin sheathing? No response. But is someone possibly remiss here? Was I becoming paranoid? Another effect of the Prednisone?

Be your own advocate or get one!

There's a difference between imagining symptoms and actual changes. Maybe not easy to discern, but don't get carried away for attention. The same as with accountants and lawyers, **you tell them** *everything* and let them deal with it. It can all be pieces to the puzzle where the expert sees a fit when others don't. But, maybe this puzzle is over *their* heads.

How much uncertainty can one take? This is me. This is what I have, compared to what I HAD! NOW, do the comparison.

I'm back to square one and to me there are no assurances. What do they care? I have to start the testing routine and delays, lack of control, yada, yada, yada, all over again? And then go down some blind alley of imaginary recovery, again, to give me hope? What right do people have to determine that I should be given "hope" or comfort with my misery, to survive in this condition instead of a choice to not survive? But in the meantime, this cruel torture of a jail cell has to be endured.

Why? Why can't a person determine when and how to end their life? Because it's a biblical taboo and only some imaginary "god" can determine when the end should come because it's said in some 2,500-year-old book that we are supposed to live for he/she/it?

C'mon, torture for some green-eyed, spaghetti bowl, imaginary, unseen, "trust me," monster-god hanging out on the other side of the moon? **We update our cellphones and computers—why not our minds?** The only thing in life that certainly shouldn't be taboo is talking about something that ALL of us are going to experience. And this becomes the crux of the problem—the perspective as to how we approach problems. During *my* "snowstorm of ill-health," I don't want hope and faith, but a cure or understanding which leads to action, if not a choice.

* * *

Now, I'm "iced." Waiting for a new diagnosis, and a maybe as to a cure, is like waiting to have a call answered when you're put on hold, or you call some office at 4:50 and the recording comes on..." Our hours are from 9am to 5 pm...." You wait, and wait, and wait, knowing that if you hang up you could have been answered the next second, or is it their end of the day and they all went home—for the night, without telling you in any way that they decided to depart early, and you're still holding. Thinking like a Dirty Harry: "Did I fire all my bullets or do I have one more left?" If I hang up... It's all relative, all some, "loop," another second on the phone, holding, could be like another 6 months. And while I'm holding or being iced, I have to endure the grip and idiocies of my body that are, by the way, getting worse for some unknown reason.

But from the age of seventy, how much time are we talking about? Like prostate cancer in men my age, doctors are not necessarily inclined to treat it. The disease will outlive the life expectancy of the patient. Well, how long am I expected to live anyway? The average for an American male is, now, about 79.6 years old. This is like playing beat the clock. Find an elixir and survive 'till you're cured, only I don't have forever to live and to enjoy that cure! Who's going to suffer the consequences if I'm pushed over the abyss waiting for a discovery and only then, maybe, a cure? Can I sign a waiver releasing them of responsibility for racing with me against the clock, regardless of the outcome? At least that's some sort of a choice!

I remember when my father was diagnosed with prostatic cancer some 45 years ago. He lived for ten more years after his diagnosis; but every day he, as well as the family, was reminded of his failing health.

It was like a slow drip of poison every day until the end when he died and I, for one, was quite relieved that the ordeal was over. No one really wants to be reminded of the daily symptoms of our misery. And I feel I'm confined to a closet in Nairobi by not being able to discuss it. I don't want that for my family. I didn't ask for the trade: Live longer but without dignity, and mental anguish for others?

In retrospect, I believe it was fortuitous that my Dad survived as long as he did. There were things about the man that I had an opportunity to realize as his testosterone decreased, and his aggression/demeanor changed. He became somewhat more of a person you could get in touch with. I don't know that I have, or want, that fortitude. But I'm sure it could be someplace.

Because I learned so much of his failings as a father, I also believe I corrected most of those chinks that he had in his armor early on and applied those lessons to rearing my own children.

They'll just have their own kinks, as I did. But perhaps I also matured in those 10 years and gained the chance to understand his view of life as well as he for mine.

* * *

Are all in the arena watching my slow demise?

I found a card on my desk with some notes on it that I apparently jotted down before visiting the internist May 2018. On the back of the card were the words reminding me to tell the doctor of my symptoms: "...restless, no sleep, cottonmouth, no taste, aches, urination issues, foggy, hand cramping, midsection numb, fingertips...." These are some of my early symptoms, and in retrospect, I was describing those of neuropathy, and maybe something else, that I mentioned to the doctor—the one that continued to prescribe Augmentin. He ignored these early symptoms that should have been a red flag to do something at THAT time of the office visit. Instead, he sent me on my way, with continued use of Augmentin, to then experience full blown liver failure on top of the pending neuropathy! Schmuck, M'f'kn, dickhead!

Meanwhile, as long as this is taking to solve my problem, I don't think anybody is in a rush to end the annuity that I provide.

It reminds me of the attorney whose son, after working for the firm for a few weeks, tells his father: "Hey dad, remember that case that has been lingering in the firm for years? Well, I settled it!" And the dad says, "Schmuck, that case put you through college!" Nothing like killing the golden calf or the cow that keeps on giving...That's the new cow named "Bob" that everyone's in line to tug on his utters. After seeing my file and walking in the door, it's Bob-the-cow with voluptuous Medicare titties being stared at by a drooling, eye-popping, *Wile E. Coyote* doctor.

17

Enough of the ranting, already.

Maybe I should sell the business. If I'm deteriorating, I don't have enough energy to come up with new ideas or recipes that a business needs. I'm basically absent, and Dee can't contribute like an entrepreneur. So, who's left to run this?

I'm losing interest in the store because there's little I can contribute other than orders.

Dee is hardly interested. She says she's following my dream. But this "dream" is paying some bills. Unfortunately, she's not able to focus because of all that's on her mind. Our life's expectations and my abilities have been altered.

Since my mobility is compromised, obviously, I can't make a recipe myself. Wally, my cook-in-charge, gets somewhat overwhelmed because he has plenty of the regular stuff to keep under control. But he has been remarkable under the circumstances. So initiating a new recipe may be out of the question. And since I can't taste or smell properly, I question my integrity or reliance when it comes to a new recipe, anyway.

I know there are things to be done in the store to maintain customers and growth. Where will the change come from if no one's around to implement it? Again, I think it could be time to either sell or step away.

That dolly I bought to decrease the need for a second delivery person could be used for me. I envision myself as a Hannibal Lecter strapped on the dolly, without a face mask. Just wheel me around the place! But why, and for what? Dump the dolly in the ocean or down the steps. Oops!

So Dee comes in and tells me a story of how our 5-year-old grand-nephew is angry with his family and wants to take the car and his 4-week-old sister to come and join "Aunt Dee's club." Fun story, but I don't think I can rely on stories like that to retire. My brain is not old enough.

Had my lumbar puncture today. A whole day for a 20-minute procedure. I ended up being turned into a maple tree in the winter, tapped for the sap. When we went to the nurse's station to check-in before the procedure, the nurse noticed my SMOKED hat (I go everywhere wearing it. Great advertising.).

She says, "I know SMOKED, do you?" Of course, we admitted ownership only to hear her rave about the brisket! Says she's been there three times, had a long conversation with me awhile back, and even sent her brother there.

She's a fan!

It just goes to show how small of a world it can be. Hearing from the public, I had a smile of pride on my face as big as a grapefruit. It's the satisfaction on people's faces that keeps me going. Why do I want to eliminate one of the few things that gives me pleasure? It certainly doesn't provide the impetus to sell.

Day 343—still waiting for the latest spinal tap and blood results from Mayo. Probably another week, at least. Last night was difficult. Seems the nights are worse than the days. Not feeling any better, but ever-so incrementally worse. I said, "who am I to have the courage or fortitude to endure this worsening affliction?" How am I doing and getting through this? I'm here now and in this condition because

I'm hanging onto some, get this, "hoped for," thread of good news that this can be reversed?

But for what?

I suppose, if I didn't have this curse, I would be on this earth, retired, and looking forward to grandkids, and a cheerleader to my sons and their families to come. Hmmm. Just doesn't seem like my style. It's not enough to keep my days filled.

I'm in some condition that defies understanding. I'm spending an unusual amount of time waiting and simultaneously deteriorating while being a UFO of symptoms in the medical annals. How far over the precipice am I going to go until I cry "Uncle" and choose to forego what most would have thought was a natural passage, with pain 'till death?

18

Mind Games

Ok, now I'm seeing a therapist. No, not *that* kind of *seeing*, as in dating. You know, seeing a therapist for the head! Dee and the boys all insisted I see one. They think I'm depressed. Time for mental transformation.

Personally, I think not. Pissed off maybe, and frustrated, but not depressed. So, now it's Tuesdays with my "Morrie." She's a lovely lady, probably a little younger than I, and Medicare still picks up the bill! So, I'm happy in that respect.

But as far as my head, I'm not sure I'm going to have any breakthroughs, discoveries, or release any repressed feelings.

I think I'm pretty honest. Which is good because if you're not going to be honest with your therapist, how are you ever going to solve any problems? It will become either a hide-and-seek treasure hunt, or a moving target. Good luck with that.

Heck! What's the possible embarrassment? I'm a human being among another 7+billion. What could be so unheard of?

I initiated our first session with the prime thought on my mind that suicide was an option if this illness didn't have an expiration date because my life expectancy was approaching. I doubted I could endure going down a blind alley, finally getting cured only to find that my time was over anyway because of natural causes. My last breath is not going to end up in a museum!

All the therapists I've seen in the last 30 years were helpful, you know. Although, it may seem like a lot, on reflection, the necessity for seeing them likely presents itself as we go through life's passages. Very helpful in navigating the concomitant issues if one is open to the exploration.

But here's the funny thing. They all have quirks or styles. Some wiggle in their seats when the time is up, others take careful notes. They're humans, too, ya know.

One of the quirks this new one has is if I become silent because I'm waiting for her response, or she wants me to say something and I have nothing to say, it becomes one of those Larry David moments. She stares at me and I stare at her, and seems like we're both waiting for the other to blink first. She says it's part of her style to let things evolve, to see what flows from my mind. But can you picture the moment? Larry squinches his lips and eyes, damned if he'll blink, and she almost does the same while they both continue their facial dance.

If or when it happens again, I'll mention the Larry David thought. Otherwise, what am I doing there?

* * *

I had an intimate conversation with Dee the other night. We discussed our lack of sex over the period of more than a year and she was curious as to whether we could try. I said I get no sensation down there and that she could knock herself out trying. But, sorry, I can't even feel my pants when trying to undo them to urinate.

Although she said I could try to stimulate her, I said, "first of all, I don't have the feelings in my hands to gauge the sensitivity." I don't want to make mashed potatoes of her private parts. Although she insisted my hands feel good to her. I do have muscle memory of the touch, but there just seems to be something missing if I don't even have what a blind man has when holding his walking cane. Try caressing something with a floppy, wet dish rag. Can you get off? Ok, maybe. Maybe I'm also a little embarrassed because my libido is zero and what can a guy fake? Nothing.

* * *

How does one go from being a vibrant, independent, individual to, almost overnight, being a dependent and worse? The world has changed for me; from a world of doing, to one of being done to, or for. Accepting what others provide is never 100% the way you want or equal to how you would do it. That takes submission and compromise—acceptance of something less in your mind.

For instance, when I was at Jesse's graduation from dental school. A humongous accomplishment for him. One, for all of us, to certainly be proud of. But once again, I'm on the receiving end, accepting whatever is given; a conflict for someone who likes to maintain some control.

A different person in a wheelchair drops a magazine and, in trying to pick it up, engages in a torturous exercise until another, more capable person, runs over to relieve her of her misery. So, one aspect of this affliction is about control.

Which means it's also about throwing up one's hands and conceding helplessness. When people stand in front of you, they don't consider that the world could be viewed by the disabled from a lower vantage point. People in wheelchairs are marginalized. We're pushed ahead of everyone, headfirst into elevators, ahead of a pack instead of alongside, face first and parked against walls, headfirst, staring at the wall, or opposite the crowd. People are always talking behind your back; in essence, we're marginalized and taken out of the conversation.

Whether it's health and physical capabilities, or financial well-being, we're no less people than those that can stand upright. As a point of fact, there's little correlation between modern humans of intelligence and their ability to stand erect.

It becomes about ceding some self-determination and occupying your own carved-out space. The disabled, in essence, become relegated to the add-ons: the quietly talked about, the concerned PC group. The "better he than I crowd" simply because we can't stand up straight or run a hundred-yard dash in less than 10 seconds!

Did we bargain for this? My family, relegated to caretakers; taking the wheelchair out, pushing me, helping with my dressing, unscrewing bottle-caps, addressing an envelope or filling out a questionnaire, and certain chores that my malfunctioning body prevents me from doing easily for myself? Now I'm controlling a large portion of her time?

I was the Dad, the one who helped THEM get dressed. It used to be fun peeling a Clementine. Now it's an exercise in frustration, trying to stay clean after dripping all over. Unfortunately, some of us have had shit thrown at us and some of it stuck. And because it wasn't our choice, we get discounted or marginalized, and thrown under some bus. But reality check: My needs as described won't end there—the longer we live, the greater the attention to meeting my needs there'll be. Who looks forward to that!

* * *

On the way to Jesse's graduation, I was disappointed with the Doctor's phone conversation concerning my need for physical therapy. Where is the science or the overwhelming number of articles about this discovery that physical therapy restores neurological sensation? None that I could find!

Not to mention the fact that Prednisone, as ubiquitously a prescribed drug as Cod liver oil years ago, also, leads to muscle breakdown and irritability.

From Northwestern's Feinberg School of Medicine:

" "One of the major problems of using steroids such as pred- *"*
nisone is they cause muscle wasting and weakness when
taken long term."

Build up muscle with rehab, then tear it down with steroids. Is this a calculated tradeoff, or a punt?

It just comes down to a matter of time—a matter of shoveling shit against the tide waiting for the inevitable. We'd be better off on a rocket ship to the sun—with or without a water bottle.

I will concede that physical therapy can aid in partial restoration of or maintenance of balance because the muscles are involved. But I don't believe any connection to restoration of nerve damage exists.

I just want to sit home, eat, and not have to be bothered with anything, except the store. Even that becomes problematic at times. I don't have the energy to pursue those hidden secrets of success that all businesses require.

I told my therapist about my Larry David chuckle and she too laughed. But imagine, she said she rarely watches the tube, no less Larry. I also went on to tell one of his predicaments when he had a single ticket for a baseball game and needed to get to the ballpark in a hurry. So, of course Larry wants to beat the traffic by taking the HOV express lane; but realizes he can't drive in that lane being the only occupant. But never fear with Larry; he picks up a hooker as a temporary passenger to be the 2nd occupant in the car. What ensues in their episode is typical curmudgeon-like banter. He's taking her off the street so what's the fee? And why, he's not requiring a full service—just an accommodation. Does he have to engage in conversation—a different kind of intercourse? You get the picture. This is how my sessions go with my gal therapist just to keep it friendly. There are plenty of other topics to occupy my time than constantly being reminded to keep checking all avenues to restoration of my health. What's that definition of "insanity," is doing the same thing over and over again expecting different results?

During my therapy session I also explained my thoughts about going emotionally from mellow to anger, 0-60, immediately. Although I have a history of getting revved up, I believe it's even more exacerbated because of the "wonder" drug, Prednisone, a steroid. Think of all the football players on steroids. They can be a mean and angry lot on the field, and it follows them off the field too. I remember a high school buddy who played college football in South Dakota and returned for a high school reunion. He was as big as a house. His name was Lyle Alzado, and he won a Superbowl ring with the Los Angeles Raiders with his intimidating style.

In his words: "I became very violent on the field and off it. I did things only crazy people do. Once a guy sideswiped my car and I beat the hell out of him. Now look at me. My hair's gone, I wobble when I walk and have to hold on to someone for support, and I have trouble remembering things." He died in 1992, at the age of 43, insisting steroids attributed to his death.

* * *

I get my IVIG starting next week. That's Intravenous immunoglobulin (IVIG). From Google: "...is a blood product prepared from the serum of between 1,000 and 15,000 donors per batch."

Starting May 28, in my home, one week a month, five applications per week, for six months, at a cost of, so I'm told, $20,000 per month. Medicare will pick up a good portion of it, but the nursing agency said that, based on need, the last $2,500 could be picked up by additional aid. Maybe that's why I wasn't blitzed with the stuff early on in the hospital—too expensive! But now ok?!

Naturally, one in their right mind would say how can I live in a nice home and not have $2,500 per month to keep you alive? First of all, maybe I'm not that interested in staying alive with what I have. So, if it doesn't entirely cure me, why should I pay for it? And secondly, if I didn't even prescribe it, why should I be expected to pay for it?

Day 359 and my hands just keep getting worse. I asked Dee if she thought I was the same now as when I got out of the hospital in October and she said, "worse." Ah Ha! So, it's not my imagination. For starters, I need two hands to hold glasses or coffee cups steady. I feel the numbness and tingling is a little more pronounced in my tongue, lips, and cheek. I'm not feeling very encouraged by my prognosis with this slowly creeping affliction. This "creature" that has a grip around me is something out of Twilight Zone. The day of my death, the moment of passing, there will be this imagined, alligator-lizard-looking creature that will dislodge itself from around me and slowly slither away, onto another unsuspecting soul.

I will not be a Head-in-the-Bed, I will not.

Had my second home infusion today. Always seems to be an adventure of some sort with this illness. The IV inserted by the first nurse a couple of days ago was somewhat faulty. It kept leaking. At one point, when 90% finished, it fell out on its own leaving a rather large hole in my skin and I.V.I.G. fluid leaking out. Ech!

Just the sight of that little hole, for some reason, was creepy. Now, a decision had to be made to either be done with this infusion and waste the 50ml. of precious remaining fluid or stick again with another IV and finish the bag of goodies. The latter was the choice and a good one.

Uneventfully, and to my surprise, the new nurse inserted the IV in the other arm, this time on top, behind the wrist, she found a vein, good enough for her. Sounds like something out of the thousand positions of the Kama Sutra. So, why did it take the first nurse three times?!

To add a little more misery, confusion, and excitement to the day, the modem for our internet was a victim of a thunderstorm. Just another issue for my Prednisone-infused brain to deal with. Brrrrrr!

And then, of course, while the store was working on getting out an order for 280 people, the smoke detector decided to sound an alarm. Guess who came to dinner? About six firemen, in full regalia, along with their trucks. False alarm. Life as usual nowadays.

* * *

I saw my lady shrink today. She liked that I referred to my adaptation to my new life as "retooling." Well, it is, to some degree, and it comes with a cost. If I could do a life-cycle analysis based on my life expectancy I would have a better idea of how to bet on my survival. Problem is, of course there are no guarantees as to one's life expectancy. On the other hand, if this condition becomes worse—who wants to live longer like this, anyway?

* * *

June 4, two days ago now, was the one-year anniversary being in this dreadful gulag of mine. I'm also getting bored of this writing and endurance. The belly's getting bigger, the body stiffer, hands still progressing to useless, if that's even possible, and the chest-vice tightening at will. If I ate one more bite, my stomach blew up beyond retraction, and exploded, hemorrhaging all over; I wouldn't care. Take me. What more tortures could be devised that could stand in the way of my wishes? How desperate a human am I that I can't act? I see tits 'n asses and I still can't act. I miss my life as remembered. I can't believe I'm in this condition. Nothing happens fast enough with this illness. Maybe nothing will happen, at all.

19

The Boys

My sons are great. Beyond indulgent. They know I need help doing things, so they are very attentive. I was showing Landon where to trim the tall corn plant the other day and while holding on to the tree, it started to tip over. Did I notice? Apparently not. Slowly I dove into the couch. A funny moment. "Hey dad—what're you doing down there?"

Jesse is just as good. Always trying to be ahead of me when getting in or out of the car, needing a cart for stability, and asking if he can go ahead to save me some steps.

Concerned about my looks, as Dee is, he wants to help with trimming my beard, straightening my clothes, and is always there. For what to do to reverse my ailment—I'm sure he feels frustrated and helpless.

Of course, I wouldn't tell them I went down, falling again, because of the low blood pressure. But I know that when they bring a glass of water to me without request, they're saying: "I love you."

Seems like, overnight, I've become my parents, aging before my time. As if I fell off of a cliff. I feel compromised, diminished, and dependent. Not a good feeling. Am I going for a tolerance award? A new example of a role-model? A PTSD sufferer? An alcohol-tamed neuro zombie? Did I do something so horrible that this is payback? I doubt it. If this IS payback, Hell can't be that much worse.

IT WAS ONLY A BOWLING BALL!

* * *

I watched a segment of Chernobyl on HBO this evening. The scene where one of the men laying in a hospital bed with the effects of radiation exposure is pathetic. He'll never recover. Looks like he had considerably more time left to his life anyway. How does that compare with what's left of mine? It would have been so much easier to administer euthanasia to the poor guy, and call it a day!

"Gee. He was just here a minute ago." –George Carlin.

My body looks horrible. The stomach is distended and sagging into something that looks like a malnourished Biafra child. The veins in my arms show the battlefield of the last twelve months of little blood sucking spears, needles and IV's of all types. The legs show flabby skin around pockets of where muscle used to be, which have withered away from little use and Prednisone. My early morning vision is blurred from the cataract surgery. It's becoming difficult to scratch an itch, if I can even feel one. The scratch just doesn't feel satisfying, the same as what feels more satisfied after a scratch, the finger, or the ear? And with the numbness becoming more intense around my waist, I can scratch and scratch and scratch, to little end.

No pleasure there. I'm not getting much pleasure anywhere. I feel like my blind and deaf dog coping with something unexplainable. Why should I be any different—because I can verbalize it? Although we make so much more of our existence because we can verbalize, are we entitled to a different perspective of that existence? Lions, horses, whales, and the rest of the animals on Earth didn't create climate change.

I walk around in a half-fog and hung-over, drug induced, stupor, wanting to take naps every few hours. Fatigue always lurks around the corner. One sufferer described her energy level as being given a ration of "spoons" every day. Morning hygiene takes 2 spoons; dressing two. Reading the morning news three. Now, when your allotment is say 12 spoons a day how many spoons remain for a day's activities. IVIG doesn't promote nerve regeneration. It may facilitate it, but nowhere do I read that it restores nerve tissue or Myelin sheathing. So, why am I bothering? I'm really just going through somebody's motions, to say, "well, we tried."

Who wouldn't be rationally depressed or suffer any other depression after living a life with full attributes and then abruptly having them taken away? Sounds like, to me, I'm a PTSD victim, to say the least.

Tell me there aren't programs administered to those who need the readjustment. War vets, automobile-accident victims, shooting incidents, and who knows what other acute circumstances there are? I have an acute onset of liver failure with accompanying, life-world-changing, Neuropathy. Tell me, and all those around me, to some degree, I wouldn't be a definition of PTSD? Why would it concern some if I refused inputting the energy for, what could be, a short period of time remaining on my life-term?

All those zippity drug commercials on the tube are actors portraying recovered, healthy people. Jeeez, what false hopes! Even a ten-year-old car probably has more residual value—not to mention, a child! Now tell me what residual value there is to a 70-year-old person with my affliction. Even roofs on houses, cars, tires, anything else with a warranty comes with a residual value. Why are people also with life expectancies and defects (illnesses) not credited with its own residual value and then afforded the opportunity to determine whether we keep the "roof" or not?

20

Do we live for a "higher authority?"

Am I out of my mind in some way? How dare I even consider taking my own life, say some. Only "He," the lord, has a right to give and take a life—right?

And if I am depressed it's certainly more "reactive" (to an event) as opposed to endogenous (a chemical imbalance from within). Maybe I don't want this roller coaster ride. I wouldn't mind drifting off in a permanently induced "sleep." That might just be No. 1 on my bucket list. My second favorite activity is probably getting into bed, at night, and letting my sleep medicine get me a good night's sleep—uninterrupted 'till morning; or maybe forever. Death with dignity. And F'k yez all, thinking you can sit in judgement!

See me as more than an old person with an illness. I'm someone blessed having experienced life. But I was also gifted the dignity of living or dying. I want the world to see me as a person with a problem and a choice, not as a problem with no choice. I cannot escape, and don't want to cede my control to some mass of strangers that won't recognize my own right to life or death.

This is a sea change moment—something earth-shaking in history to recognize that people should have an individual right to determine under what circumstances we have to live with. Many want to control how and when we give birth, what "phantasmagorical stories" are taught in school to our children, and also extends to under what circumstances we live and die—regardless of the financial and emotional burdens attached. For one thing, how is that less government?

21

And Who wants to carve the Turkey

Day 372 and seeing my Neuro Doctor today—one week after IVIG. Not expecting any miracles—since I certainly don't feel any miraculous changes. And how can anyone tell me what to expect when they can't feel what I feel?

Not good news from him, and as I suspected. But at least I got some answers. The IVIG is for antibodies; perhaps to wash out the rogue antibody still apparently present as indicated by the elevated protein level in my spinal fluid. More to the point, to introduce new antibodies to ward off potential infection. Dr. V. will prescribe at least two more months of the treatment to see if there's any benefit to continuing. Maybe at some time, change drugs; maybe back to Rituximab. More poo on the walls.

But if the rogue cell escaped the drug the first time around, what would be different this time? Or did the new rogue cell develop after the treatment? Seems like I've been around this bush before. And I'm getting tired of chasing my tail while dragging along my entourage of difficulties... Why are the chronically unhealthy and aged doomed to follow some dead-end tortured script while we're following nature's gameplan that's worked so well for millions of years?

* * *

If there's still a presence of another culprit, it could still be destroying the protective coating, not to mention nerves; rendering any treatment moot until the destroyer is eradicated. Although the advancement of the neuropathy could one day be arrested, what gets me back to square one and in how much time, before I expire of natural causes? And is there even a square one to return to? Or is it all wishful thinking and the myth of "hope" to keep some going in search of a mythical cure—regardless of cost? A Don Quixote, fighting these imaginary windmills? Every doctor's findings becomes a new calibration of what could be wrong with me. But, so far, all a dead end. Maybe we're just not there yet.

After dwelling on my doctor's follow-up visit, it's clear that this has been a woefully mismanaged illness. From not eradicating the initial lung virus; to overdosing Augmentin and setting off the liver failure. Then not identifying and arresting the pending neuropathy, scattershot applying IVIG, rituximab, plasmapheresis in a hospital directed by a physician who had little clue.

Even declaring "good news" in believing the LGi1 was the only rogue antibody. There should have been a follow-up test to confirm that all rogues were eliminated or that I'm in a stable condition! Or forewarn me that Neuropathy can advance.

And denying the patient's "feelings" as to the progression of the illness? If this illness is unchartered waters, the patient is the main and lead alert mechanism.

It may be becoming a little clearer now, in hindsight. The residual result of my affliction, neuropathy, I have been in the wrong place. They should have recognized that fact rather than look at me like some medical giving-tree or the ever-giving cow.

Starting with "Dr. Double-down Augmentin," this is an obvious case of an avoidably innocent but ignorant drug induced iatrogenic disease starting with my liver. "Iatrogenic" is a mistake, or malpractice. It happens often. Something that can be avoided with a central database red-flagging their use of medications for conflicts and dosage.

At one time many could be taking a dozen medications. Now add to that some processed packaged food and we become human test tubes. Who knows what witches brew could be coursing through my veins? Iatrogenic is just a euphemism for "Toxic Avenger." After taking as many chemicals as a sewer, I went in as some toxic avenger and came out as "meek Melvin the mop boy."

If bombs can be made from fertilizer, I can't imagine the unintended combinations and consequences to our bodies from hosting the enormous amounts of chemical components intermingling between medications and many of our foods and environment.

From Dovepress in the National Center for Biotechnology Information:

> "*According to the World Health Organization, iatrogenic disease may be defined as adverse drug reactions or complications induced by nondrug medical interventions. In addition, iatrogenic disease has been defined....as a disease induced by a drug prescribed by a physician, after a medical or surgical procedure.*" "*Multiple medications (polypharmacy) that transform the elderly into living "chemistry sets," are probably the most ubiquitous threats for iatrogenic disease.*" "*...A recent meta-analysis (according to NIH) showed the incidence of iatrogenic disease to be between 3.4% and 33.9%.*"

Yikes! Although that's a huge discrepancy, it's certainly indicative of the unwieldy magnitude of the problem! It's hardly uncommon to take a medication for one illness and develop, say, a urinary tract infection (UTI), as a side-effect, from the urinary retention caused by the medication for the illness. Now, do we take another med to counteract the retention and the UTI infection or change the original prescription that caused the UTI retention? This part of medical procedure is not an exact science and can lead to confusion and many unrelated issues.

Our current health-care system is supported by the concept of profit-motivated capitalism, brought to us by the likes of those drug manufacturers who gave us Thalidomide of 1960's, Opioids, or dubious claims from Elizabeth Holmes' *Theranos*; or faulty medical devices like the rejected silicone breast implants of 2009; or a kidney transplant racket in India 2008; the countless ordinary examples of over-billing by physicians, hospital practices, and insurance providers.

From: *The NY Times:* "Hospitals and Insurers Didn't Want You to See These Prices. Here's Why:"

> " *"It shows hospitals are charging patients wildly different* " *amounts for the same basic services: procedures as simple as an X-ray or a pregnancy test." "...This secrecy has allowed hospitals to tell patients that they are getting "steep" discounts, while still charging them many times what a public program like Medicare is willing to pay. And it has left insurers with little incentive to negotiate well. The peculiar economics of health insurance also help keep prices high."*

And to add insult to injury, most of the entire system is supported by politicians being lobbied by the respective businesses maintaining the status quo.

It's called "the fox minding the hen-house." The system is wrong with all the interests competing for private and tax-payer dollars. Shit doesn't *"just happens"* if there's a pattern—when the condition is recognized as systemic and becoming normal. But don't just limit the accusation: think the Enrons, Tycos, HealthSouths. Think scandals. Who benefits most from excessive testing, drug administration, product promotions, and development of facilities? A single payer system with technological assistance can buy in-bulk; whether it's equipment, services, supplies, or medicines; for the benefit of society. Sick people shouldn't have to compete with profit-motivated entrepreneurs; particularly those who get the tax breaks in their bank accounts vs. those who can't even afford maintaining a family. The greed of unbridled, capitalism besmirches the credibility of the profession and the industry.

But don't doctors, pharmaceutical companies, insurance companies, and legislators all have a part in this quagmire-ignoring-Nature condition? Could it be possible that our culture of taking medication too liberally as promoted by the industry: doctors, pharmaceutical companies, advertisers on tv, and all the rest who have a self-interest in sustaining such a profitable environment? A practice which actually leads to much of our misery? Just think of the opioid epidemic for one instance. Iatrogenic for others. We're being duped.

Maybe our mentality of extending life at all costs is contrary to sustainable, Mother Nature. And could it ultimately be determined that unbridled capitalism may be good for ingenuity and inventions but not all good for society as a whole. Think greed. Think how do we fix this? It may take a sea-change in thinking and behavior. If we can sue the energy industry for climate change and injuring our environment, why not sue the medical industry for a disastrous living mentality? That's some can of worms when we think about it.

It's not about pointing one finger at the mismanagement of my case. This is about pointing 10 fingers at the elements that created a "perfect storm" for my avoidable condition. This could be a class action in reverse! I've got 3000+ pages of hospital documentation and 18 months and counting of Doctor's records. In that time no one made a mistake?! The more moving parts to a system is a greater susceptibility to failure of the system. We were grappling with an octopus of potential failures.

I think we have the "smoking gun" that indicts that pernicious and nefarious system as to even unintentional or collateral issues. Convince me I'm the only schmuck this has happened to and throw this book away!

Within six months of being discharged from the hospital, we requested the files of all the physicians who treated my condition starting with the cough in Dec. '17 leading to my admission to the hospital in June '18. Although no one thought to look much further than treating symptoms as reported, like ordering a chest cat scan because the cough was not going away. Apparently, coughs are "only" due to microbes and nothing else could be wrong. But, upon review of the files there were indications that some docs either "heard" wrong or they made things up!

One doctor said I had indications of COPD and I reported nausea and vomiting. Really? NO! But if I had, then what was the follow up? None that I could figure out.

But the major culprit in my eyes and mind, is the one who prescribed not only Augmentin again, but when he didn't see results the first time, doubled down on the dosage in spite of reported symptoms indicating the onset of neuropathy! "Let's just throw more shit at the wall and see what sticks." Didn't he see the memo regarding excessive use of Augmentin?

And if he didn't see the memo, what IS the procedure for the medical community acknowledging a potentially life and death update? To make matters worse, the doctor apparently also ignored the increased white blood count and the raised Bilirubin level which was highlighted and indicated in the bloodwork that he ordered; only to then continue with the dosage??

Piece of shit amateur, backwoods, hillbilly F'kn' doctor, who, because of his ignorance, changed my life forever. But don't think I'm angry because of what some may now think is a little-too-late, revelation to me. M-Fkr! I wouldn't want your money if you knew what you were doing at the time, and it wouldn't be necessary because this couldn't have happened. But for ending my life as I knew it and what was promising to me, and my family, I want all that's yours and your insurance company's to be mine, because you're pretending to be a licensed f'kn physician. AND if you actually are licensed, where and how did you get your license—Macy's bargain, f'kn basement? Venting over. Feelings not.

Nobody really has any clue on how to treat this beast of an illness, other than, possibly, managing pain and discomfort. More crap being thrown against me to see what sticks. A little better than a medieval application of sorcerer's remedies with the same results. Blood washing—yech! And if any of the millions have found relief from any related prescriptions, you've escaped from a burning building.

It's finally hitting home to me. This *is* serious, as I'm no longer the invincible, young at heart or mind, person anymore. The boy who never stopped growing up. But that's my business. THAT got changed practically overnight through no fault of my own. I relied on and placed my confidence in the ability of the medical system to know the operative procedure in a case like mine. But the components of the system had no clue as to what the protocol should be because it was distracted by profit and hubris. Humility was not in their playbook. Little did I realize that the medical community was dealing with a known mysterious illness. This was all new, inexperienced, territory for them.

For starters, I believe it's a result of our medical system—no central command to oversee what's being administered to a patient to prevent duplication of expensive and unnecessary procedures. The complexity of medical treatment has progressed since the days of the rural country doctor. The medical system demands a new review procedure. Fix it!

"Time heals all wounds," as the adage goes.

Apparently, it doesn't. This is not like getting a broken arm fixed where we learn to rely on tried-and-true methods, or even fighting cancer where one can have a limited statistical trust that they'll either enter remission or an outright defeat of the disease, if not death. Currently, mine is an unwinnable war with an indeterminate course, except for the ultimate disposition...

I'm actually stunned. On one hand, is this my fate? The beginning of my end? This is the outline of the script for my final days? I suppose when someone is handed the end of their life in playbook form, do they just plan accordingly? Do they even have a choice when they don't desire to follow that script? Especially when their choice is limited by the very hidden nature of the illness.

Now, what's my plan? I have a head, but the body is uncooperatively, dragged along, attempting a roadblock at every intersection of choice. This is my retirement? I can't give up yet! Or can I?

I fit into a sizable group that exists beyond the edge of help. It really is peripheral neuropathy for me. I live tightly wrapped in mummies' cloth around my limbs, around my torso, up to my neck, in a shell surrounded by the affliction with my internal organs, now blindly, going about their day as if almost nothing were wrong. My gut, feeling like someone is squeezing the shit out of me. I, alone, can't rise up and defeat my oppressive illness. The handwriting is on the wall. My hand reaching out to be saved. But I can't be the only one to experience this.

Hasn't anybody ever written about suffering from neuropathy, and its related issues, in novels or literature, other than promoting some questionable product or treatment? Has nobody complained in history, journals or their love letters, their memoirs, or even in hieroglyphics, about this affliction?

There's, obviously, no way I'm the first to write or talk about this ailment. The internet is loaded with related comments on blogs and websites. But who were the first persons to write about this hobbling, debilitating condition in real-time? Who was the first to notice this strange unexplainable illness? Did Tolstoy, Hemmingway, some Pharaoh or a Caesar complain of these symptoms? How did they describe it? What were their first attempted treatments? How did they cope? Is there a history other than late 19th or 20th century recognition of the symptoms, or mention that Queen Anne of Great Britain, and cousin King Henry VIII could have had the affliction related to their, believed-to-have, diabetes? Is there a thread of connectivity anywhere? Maybe my neuropathy was a result of environmental conditions only as presently known. Or did I eat too much buttered popcorn as a child?

And what's so different about getting a leg cut off? For one, I could get a prosthesis. Suppose I had Myasthenia Gravis or the likes? It would grow on me and I would have time to adjust. Suppose I got killed or became a paraplegic from a car accident? The former would put me out of my misery. The latter has the same dilemma based on age. But what are the stories that follow the others with my same predicament? The stories and feelings that haven't, as yet, been heard. Is living under any condition the demanded tradeoff for life?

To some, it may be. But not all want the trade. There are millions of sufferers in one form or another, each with their own tolerance.

22

Father's Day, Empty Nest

Father's Day was yesterday. That was a great day, regardless of my circumstances. I was reminded that a year ago I was in the hospital passing out with nurses calling code blue.

So, we had surf and turf this year with close friends sharing our feast.

It's been two years since my last enjoyable summer. One summer never happened, the other was taken away. I don't know if there's even a justifiable and fair comparison. But nowadays, I do have a lot of time on my hands, and different things do come to mind.

I sit outside on my deck in the rear of the house. It's all secluded, surrounded by trees, very lush and full. All very quiet except for the rustling of the wind. It's the quiet dusk that precedes my uneventful evening. I think it could be my last summer here. Either the house gets sold, or maybe I'm not hobbling around this earth anymore. It's a cruel and painful punishment being acutely afflicted and directionless like this.

Unless there's significant improvement in my condition and I'm still here, then I'm really talking up a big game of BS. Or I just don't have the balls to do myself in. After all, I still have my head, both eyes, and, apparently, I just don't want to give it up or give in to it, yet. Maybe I'm just a novice when it comes to self-execution.

A worm doesn't complain, why should I? The kids are leaving, Dee and I are empty nesters. She wants an easier life. And although I want to be more relaxed, I fear I'll be bored alone and with my computer, just waiting. We have less to talk about—she's one for the phone or texting.

But although I can think about committing suicide, it hardly means one will actually follow up. How do we get to that moment, when doing the act will actually mean the end?

Surely a person must be in significant pain to even consider the act so as not to want to see tomorrow. But how does one know what that pain threshold is as prerequisite for completing the act? Am I in a burning building with the flames licking at me and I'm compelled to jump? The pain threshold is different for all, and justifiably so. How do we equate the two when both are clearly in pain but no way to compare?

How does one pick the style and method when they arrive at their end? I suppose I wouldn't pick a violent method. It would hurt, no? Hari-kari, jumping off a building, crashing the car... Not to mention the f'kng mess and consequences after. I don't want to impose.

And suppose the chosen method didn't work? Then I could be worse off and really be a head-in the-bed. Drowning? How do you stay down that long before you want to gasp for air? Pills...What's the prescription and dose to get it done? My luck I'll be in a coma from an underdose or overdose. Then what did I accomplish? And then who deals with it? Think of people chaotically, self-medicating.

If these methods fail, then I'm still trapped in my cage. What is the method that will leave less for the insurance company to question, if there can even be a question about the insurance company sentencing someone to a fate like this because they may deny a suicide claim? I bought the insurance when I was healthy. Now, I'm not. What's to disqualify?

What's that about the Eighth Amendment? "...nor cruel and unusual punishments inflicted." If I had rats crawling into my coffin-of-a-cell, eating me alive, and I decided to self-terminate by poking my eyeball with my finger, and piercing my brain, would the hastening of my demise not be acceptable? Denying benefits because someone was compelled to live a life of torture to satisfy some covenant is beyond cruel and unusual punishment. Let's get real. Do they realize that my plight of survival equates to continued duress, or torture? Would I be out of my mind to want to take my life? Gee, then I must be ill and suffering mental illness. Or looking at it another way: So, Medicare pays to keep us alive so the life insurance company doesn't have to pay a claim? Wouldn't that, too, be a can of worms? And then there'll certainly be something else to talk about. Paging Larry David.

How is this situation simplified so we can stop relegating people to torture because healthy people can't make up their minds to determine the fate of the tortured? How about self-determination over one's body? Also sound familiar?

* * *

My family is big on me using pot for my symptoms. First of all, whenever smoking weed when younger, I would get somewhat paranoid. And the last time, a few years ago, while Dee and I were on vacation in Negril, Jamaica, I had the local Ganja-infused brownies. It was after that experience that I knew why some people never come home. "Oh, he's found another life among the Rastafarians."

I still get paranoid, but less so with the kids and wife. I mean, if one can't be relaxed with family, who's left, just another pothead? But on my first return foray with pot, I was a little apprehensive. For years, we had to hold our children in check, away from its usage because it was illegal.

But with all the latest hoopla, it's hard to "fight the tape." So, our youngest, having gone to school in Vermont, is the family's proponent. Not pushing it per se but exposing some of the myths we carry around from our less informed teenage days.

And the statistics coming from the now legalized states, bears out some of the misconceptions and new realities of dealing with the substance; weighing the benefits vs. the drawbacks.

My first observation is that the pot and quantities of THC, the hallucinogenic substance that gets one "high," exceeds the concentration from the pot that we smoked while growing up. So, all usage, I guess, should be recalibrated when going from one 1970's sample to the current stuff. Whereas sharing a joint with a friend years ago would be barely enough to satisfy the urge, today one toke is plenty.

Although the usage was intended to relieve my symptoms, I have to say that the laughter that it promoted was enough to forget some of my troubles. I like to laugh, but I doubt that I can walk around always giddy and high, and laughing that much until my side hurt. Or maybe I can. Opioids anyone? That was fun!

And then there's the CBD usage, the chemical substance that many believe holds the magic elixir to recovery from all of humankind's diseases and sufferings without getting the THC or the high attributed to smoking pot. The problem is that dosages vary. It often must be used in greater amounts than what's available over the counter and can get quite expensive for an experiment to try to get the right quantities and strain of CBD.

Since I'm a science-based guy, if there's no science to back up the hype, then I become a skeptic. And a final reason for not becoming a fan, is that cannabis is still considered a class one drug in the US. That means one can still be arrested on a federal level.

It also means that legitimate scientific testing and gathering of statistics to its use is hardly available because the substance itself is prohibited—so how do you get it to experiment with? There should be a debate about the legalization of pot at least for experimentation. We do it with all other drugs; why is this different? Maybe big pharma or the alcohol companies have a problem with more competition? So what? The Capitalistic system says it's ok to fail when a better or progressive mousetrap replaces another. But oh, big pharma employs a lot of people; "too big to fail?" Feel like a dog chasing its tail...?

For now, all I can do is: "I get by with a little help from my friends." (and family). And, for what it's worth, 10mg of THC with 1mg CBD, state-dispensed lozenges, an hour before bedtime, is enough to help me get a decent night's sleep.

Truncal neuropathy is like a spasm or muscle tightness that won't relax. Yet perception of a contraction of the muscles into an ever-gradual tightening, vise-like grip, completely around the torso must really be an illusion. Although it feels like a medieval body armor made of fine metal mesh, actually, I believe the nerves are misfiring or stuck in gear fantasizing that the muscles are tightening when they're not. Yet when I lay still and flinch my torso muscles, it feels like two magnets are similarly opposing each other and repelling the like poles. Feels rippley, weird, and exhausting.

So now after 13 months, what do I have to show for this as progress or improvement?

Zilch.

As a matter of fact, I look like a junkie. I've actually gone backward. Things are still getting worse, and why?! Because obviously there's no urgency since I'm now just a number in the system. There's no cure, or apparently any for that matter. Thanks, maybe, for spending a shitload of money on drugs and testing, and for some people on trying, but improvement ain't happening. Yet, hey, what do I know? I'm just the patient. The diver alone in a diving bell.

* * *

At some point this squeaky wheel is going to make a lot of noise. On the other hand, I could eventually grind down the family because I'm going to be ever more dependent. I could also disappear into the system, just showing up for checkups, maintenance, and the ultimate status report. Can you imagine if I decided to visit a doctor every time I had a new complaint from the illness or adverse medication interaction because we're all in unchartered territory? That gets pretty expensive, time consuming, and debilitating, searching in the wilderness. And I'm sure this doesn't only happen to me.

From a letter I sent to my two neurologists:

"...I WOULD LIKE TO BE CONSIDERED AS A CANDIDATE FOR WHAT-EVER TESTING IS AVAILABLE—APPROVED OR NOT, TO IDENTIFY AND ELIMINATE THIS NEW ANTIBODY... I AM READY TO VISIT THE MAYO CLINIC AGAIN, OR WHEREVER, FOR TREATMENT, ASAP...."

That note of desperation, apparently, fell on deaf ears. But as things are now, what could they do?

* * *

My sister came from Florida to visit. I think it was about two years ago since we last saw each other. So, obviously she hasn't seen me in my condition. But she had a lot to offer regarding our mother's health in her final years. Apparently mom also suffered from neuropathy of the feet. It was this condition that persuaded her to stop driving. Immediately, the question comes to mind, is it hereditary? And was I present, but not tuned in to my mother's other complaints when she, too, was perhaps, also, suffering from this nasty ailment? Originally, she was diagnosed with Myasthenia Gravis; until upon further thought—she wasn't. The more I think back on her complaints, I believe I'm not far behind.

Aging is largely hereditary. Humans come with a large variety of potential failings of their moving parts. Some succumb to their maladies; others get their illnesses successfully treated. That's really what we're doing with medicine. Now how do we look at ourselves? For years we believed we were created and dictated to by Gods. Now we need a new, updated, way of thinking. Although we may be on the top of the food chain, we're still part of the animal kingdom. Why do we deserve special treatment from the rest?

23

The Isle of Boiling Frogs

Today's temperature is about 85 degrees and I got dizzy—light-headed, really. But I also became disoriented, not knowing what day it was or what time I had an appointment later in the day. This was scary to me. Is this the start of something to come, or just a transient issue related to heat? I doubt there can be any definitive answers.

I've become momentarily forgetful or disoriented, not knowing for a few moments where I'm driving to in the car. While driving, I sometimes forget what street I'm on or where I'm going. Distinguishing certain images becomes confusing for a few moments; Maybe due to executive processing issues?

Too coincidental to pass it all off as to age-related. I can have a thought in my mind one second and forget it the next. I just want to curl up and go to sleep. I even mistake crawl for curl and other similar spelling mistakes.

> "Apparently a year after IVIG, Robert could not expend the energy hoping and waiting—going down a road to nowhere. Like a simmering pot needs a little energy to maintain the simmer, Robert's energy level dropped below that minimum to keep him alive. He lost his simmering enthusiasm for life."

-My likely obituary at this point.

Bohemian Rhapsody and living longer. What am I going to be missing by living longer—all the reruns and do-overs? The next LeBron; Episode 19 of *Star Wars*; the melting of the polar ice-caps?

Kk—I get it. I'd be missing all the real-time stuff—like the same grandkids growing up and the usual ice-cream and cake along the way; and maybe even the 2052 elections! But there's a big price to pay for the opportunity and privilege of life. My father passed away before meeting any of my children and they couldn't be finer. What could be different? My job was completed with raising my kids. That's what nature intended. Job done.

My stirpes can be proud to continue nurturing the Feuerstein name and genes to come.

I can make sure I get candle number one at the Bar/Bat Mitzvah candle lighting ceremonies. So when Rachel, Roxanne, Ralph or Ratzo Rizzo light candle number one for Gpa Rob, I will live on, surrounded by tears forever-more. Sort of like the annual 9/11 memorials. Well, maybe I'm being presumptuous.

Now I'm on Cymbalta, and as prescribed by the doctor, I also have urinary issues to deal with. I've also had a couple of visits with the new psychiatrist. You know, the one who's going to "treat" my depression.

What a joke. The first time, I saw the nurse practitioner who took my vital info and prescribed my continuance of Amitriptyline but doubled the dosage. So, I took an extra pill from my normal dosage of 10mg at night and I was loopy the next day. I realized it wasn't great for me to be in a stupor, so I discontinued the increased dosage. Besides, I would, soon find out that doubling a dosage wasn't the brightest idea for Amitriptyline and the accompanying urinary issues. More failures in the system.

They're using paraprofessionals for real doctor's work, attempting to cut costs. But who's going to pay for their failures? The for-profit doctor's practice saves the money and reaps the savings. The patient pays for the mistake. Give me a real doctor, not the bullshit practice so they can increase profits by employing paraprofessionals. Should health care be contingent on profit? There's a tug-of-war going on here between the profit from increased revenues and the sensibility of more accurate managed care.

After my visit with the new neurologist in the city, she also preferred me to be on Cymbalta because it was not only an antidepressant, it also helped with the effects of the neuropathy pain and, if at all possible, nerve regeneration. Problem is that the Cymbalta made it difficult to urinate. So, the pain and excruciating discomfort is not worth the unconfirmed healing properties. More to muddle through. I'll stop taking it altogether and avoid possible iatrogenic side effects.

But here's the thing, when I went back the second time for the psych-shrink visit, the waiting room was filled and I was told there were a couple of patients ahead of me. So, my being on time to a shrink would mean that two people ahead of me would be maybe an hour and a half wait by typical shrink time. Only, hold on—the two that were ahead of me were out in 15 minutes, and when I was called, my visit lasted a mere 7 minutes or so. Did the doc even ask about my mental condition or suicidal thoughts? Of course not.

I, too, was out with a new prescription phoned into the pharmacist for Cymbalta in no time.

This was not a psych practice to vent one's frustrations, but a drug-mill for prescriptions. This guy was a revolving door and if some think I was going to be a part of it, they're mistaken. I'm not some Oxycontin-type drug addict, despite trying to find some relief for an incurable disease. So, I'm going to take these medications and be one happy asshole for some other's comfort and profit, and endure the side effects to boot; particularly when the benefits just don't outweigh the inconvenience?

My choice. No deal!

Now, I understand how people get "hooked" on opioids. Few people ask the questions. But who are those patients willing or capable to challenge the system of, among other things, questioning the doctors?

On top of that, I have my third application of IVIG next week. Whoopee! Unfortunately, I don't see any improvement on that front, either. I'm just going through the motions, being milked and enabled by what's available in the system. This is why Medicare busts the bank. Thanks for the effort, but it doesn't seem like anything's working; and at some point, I'll say, "No more. Don't waste your money. I've crossed over that bridge to the island of slow-boiling frogs, to eventually go where all unsuspecting frogs go because there's little to do anyway.

* * *

I just found out that my autonomic reflex test that I've been waiting for since March is now scheduled for the end of October. Some urgency—right? I could be dead—but wait six months? I'd have longer than you know who to resurrect myself!

I'm subtly getting the hint, delivered with the impact of a sledgehammer. My affliction is a losing battle. And, with that, I'm quietly getting the message that I have permanent damage, or at least the damage will outlive my life expectancy. Give it up and resign myself to the prognosis—futility. But maybe I'm understanding that those Opioid addicts are really just intentionally ending their lives with their drugs. Their suicide wish. Who's fooling whom? Ignorance is blissful? Maybe some users aren't as dumb as we think?

If I cut myself deeper everyday, one could witness the progress of the cut or the healing of the damage. But the only thing anyone can see when looking at me is my blown-up, extended belly, and my physical movements. Otherwise, why would anyone other than a doctor testing my body be aware that something is wrong?

But by just sitting down and speaking, all appearances are healthy and there's little indication that something's amiss. That's, reportedly, the guilt-promoting part of this illness. Those who feel others, not seeing the likes of a leg amputated, that this population of sufferers are fabricating their illness. But just watch me and other neuromuscular challenged sufferers try to open a medicine dispenser whose pills are meant to combat our illness or those damn plastic food containers. Desperation will be the end of us hopelessly trying to prove our invisible disease. And leftovers will become a thing of the past because opening those damn containers is next to impossible.

Day 410 "...Currently, I think he is in good hands, based on my last call with them [local doctors], although he has a difficult problem." Another one raises the white flag. "...he has a difficult problem."

This was the profound two-line response from the letter written by the Mayonnaise Clinic Wizard to my son's Dr. V and Dr. K. Apparently, I've moved my slot from number 500 on someone's list to possibly one-of-a-kind.

Why couldn't a professional just say it in English, "It doesn't look good. You're fucked."

Instead, I'm tethered to their hook. Let's keep tinkering. How many times can we keep looking under my hood? Now I understand the "no urgency to seeing me or prescribing something rehabilitative." The bomb went off and we're dealing with the rubble.

No, we're not. There is no we, and I alone will live in the rubble forever, until I don't.

Am I pissed and sad? Sure. But I have to also remind myself that regardless of the possible missed opportunities, there are people suffering from the likes of Parkinson's, Myasthenia Gravis, Guillain–Barré, who are basically in a similar situation as I, or worse, and also have little control over their prognosis.

So, should I be accepting of my condition? I just fall into the category of the unknown. Just another discombobulation of medical symptoms. If this illness is threatening the late-stage part of my life, there must be a way to foil its resolve that leads to my discomfort. Instead of chasing my tail in search of a nonexistent cure, there's got to be a way to outsmart my invisible opponent. I have the answer.

I reluctantly and skeptically started my third session of IVIG this week, day 411 into this ordeal. What is this supposed elixir? The whole process is already tiresome and tedious. Facebook groups with people suffering illnesses similar to mine only point out the futility of combating the illness with minimal success. How does one undo a curse?

Spartacus or any of my other childhood heroes would be proud. Even my dad would probably be amazed, although living with prostatic cancer for ten years, it wasn't with the difficulty of wiping one's butt and all the other symptoms encompassed by this disease. And I don't know if it's my imagination, but I get the feeling that every time they mutsher with my body, something changes the numbness or stiffness to make me believe they worsened it... I just dunno. Who does? Nobody has sufficient answers. I feel like a Lewis and Clark Expedition. Who knows what lay ahead?

I'm also not sure I'll advocate, anymore, for the "at-home care." Although on paper it has all the indications and promises of comfort and convenience, I'm not sure it has the expertise, dependability, or professionalism of a hospital or clinic.

Maybe I can watch TV, go to the fridge for a snack, or the bathroom is a shorter trip, cleaner, and more private, at home. And yea, I get to sleep a little later. But the same comforts are available in the infusion centers, with more dependability but without the additional safety concern of allowing a stranger into your home. Now, I may be being somewhat cruel here because visiting-nurses are all licensed and why should there be any negatives? But should they encounter a problem, such as inserting an IV, time becomes wasted waiting for backup to come, if it ever does at all. Consequently, whereas a backup nurse or a boss could be a half-hour or more away, in a hospital, a backup could easily be down the hall and ready to jump on.

Another downside to home care is that these nurses are practically treated like cleaning ladies and these infusions are really administered by home-care contractors. All motivated by profit, of course.

Sure, nurses are the ones who do the work, but the service is like a contractor who "subcontracts" out the work to a pool of nurses who may have an open schedule that day.

So, the problem is really communication and responsiveness of the pool. A hospital on the other hand has the pool, in-house, and can schedule in advance whereas the home-care almost waits until the last minute to confirm. Who has the patience?

My application of IVIG can be time and volume sensitive. If I want to speed up the application and shorten the number of days to say three or four, then each session will have to be lengthened to account for the greater volume applied in the shorter time. Another consideration could be installing a "port" so that the IV could come out after the use and then the port just reentered on the next application. The port accepts the needle on a regular basis without consideration of waring out a tissue puncture. As a patient, who wants to think about such things? So, after this fourth application, I'm signing up with the hospital or an infusion center the next time around. I want service.

With my mental outlook lately, I'm ambivalent about the whole thing. If I died tomorrow, I don't think I'd care! I've lost maybe 90% of my muscle and I'm 70. I'm not going to restore anything like what I've lost. I mean, who is this all for when I have to be the one enduring all the pain and inconvenience? For who's benefit am I being kept alive in my condition?

Currently. I have a dream about my restaurant and a food truck. That's what really gets me up in the a.m. Believe it or not, not my family. My love for them is categorical. But it should be my choice. My obsession for accomplishing a business is self-consuming while distracting me from the rain.

At this point I'm only driven because I'm not ready to find the courage or method that ends my suffering, but possibly more that my interest is piqued to see some resolution to a legal remedy.

When I looked into possibly pursuing legal action, I was told that the laws prevent frivolous lawsuits. Unless you can point a finger at someone and say, "He did it," you don't have a case or a chance. They say, "shit happens."

I'll tell you what shit happens, when a patient sues a doctor because he isn't current on the application of the drug that has ruined countless lives. Nothing the medical community can do will restore me to my prior self. But how about maybe eliminating law-suit protection against malpracticing doctors when something as blatant as my case arises and we shouldn't have to second guess procedures?!

Dee takes an issue with how negative I can be. Really? Is there something positive that I've missed to tip my scales? Trade places with me for only 5 minutes, let alone 400 days and still, relentlessly, counting.

My fingers can't separate but get caught in everything. I walk like a drunken sailor? How about like a spastic cripple, polio victim, without a cane, an IV stuck in my arm, and the fingers as numb and working like the little crane in an amusement park, only, I'm playing 24/7 trying to grab a prize. Maybe holding toilet paper without incident would be prize enough for me. Note to self: 2-ply toilet paper works best and keep the fingernails short—if ya know what I mean. Is this diminution in my quality of life the trade-off for living longer? Where do we draw the line? Help. I'm not really interested in exploring my tolerance level.

I'm bruised and banged up all over because I uncontrollably bump into things. Wall-hangings hang at their peril because I'm indiscriminate when I'll lurch forward or backward and successfully reach the unintended target. I won't even try to rehang them dare I do more and worse damage. I go from: who I was, to who I am, or even who am I? Try again to convince me why I can't be negative in light of the latest behavior and findings. There's far more of the negatives to deal with than the positives in getting a little more time on this earth. This one you'll just have to trust me.

In the beginning of my hospital journey, maybe I should have been relocated to a facility that focuses and is more familiar with my affliction instead of some old-time neurologist wanting to "play" the part of an immunologist.

My belly's so big, someday, I'll be asked to play that cartoon dinosaur character, Earl Sinclair. I'll probably die of a blown-up belly before something related to my neuropathy. Could that work to end my misery?

Too bad Dee doesn't get it. I'm not in the same place as she is. She wants me to wear a collared shirt and pants to match. "I look better." But I can't be bothered with my appearance anymore. And if I don't respond according to her script or likes? Too bad. My plate is full.

Cut someone some slack as they see their last days with some happiness before them. Sounds dramatic? Nice sentiment. But, **Priorities change.** You, too, trade places with me. You'll see what's important. I've entered another life.

Day 422 and here's hope for ya. My son Bryce has been in contact with the Precision Medicine Institute connected with the University of Alabama. He recently read an article on how they're using Artificial Intelligence to investigate exotic diseases on the molecular level.

So, this could be a longshot to arrest the progression of the affliction, if the unidentified, rogue protein could be identified and eradicated, but as of now, little benefit to nerve regeneration, and not in my lifetime.

* * *

As the air of a cool summer evening gently rolls across my arms, I realize this is my heaven, sitting on the backyard-deck after dinner. Unfortunately, it is not to last long.

Yesterday, as I got out of the car, and stood for a few moments, my knees buckled and down I went. I sprained my knee.

This is not fun, nor am I thrilled for my future.

24

Catering to the Masses

Catering at the store has been busy. If not for that, what would be my purpose or have something that's interesting? What would push me? What would occupy my time?

It's called a distraction. I can't imagine sitting around and just looking at something on the internet. If I can't do something constructive, I doubt that a complacent life would suit me. I can't even get lost on a golf course! Am I supposed to be happy that someday, maybe, I might see grandchildren or wait for a visit or phone call from the boys? That's not realistic or a way to conduct one's life, waiting. Other people have their lives to live without expecting them to always be there for only me.

The other day Dee remarked that "her husband was taken." Or she lost her husband. I can't remember the exact words, but I agree. I may be physically here, but for one thing, we lost the intimacy that we shared and kind of expected as we aged.

I hold on to whatever dignity I can. I had two hot dogs for dinner tonight. And I made them. Well maybe not quite two. One slipped out of the bun and tried to escape across the floor. I don't know where it went. It didn't tell me. But our dog has a Cheshire-cat grin on her face. I'll report the hot dog MIA and the dog's cat-like behavior.

* * *

I fell again. Or, as I coined it, "a controlled fall." And this time I shed a tear, or two. I know something's not right, and I'd rather my boys not see me in this condition of deterioration and need. I don't think it'll get better. This is not a way for them to remember their father. Remember me for my good days, not the ravaged end by an uninvited alien.

We sometimes treat our pets with more respect than humanity. My dog, Savanna, now downstairs in the mud room because she's defecating all over. So, we're treating the symptoms and containing it. Just like treating me. Some would use a diaper or put a mat on the floor (for the dog, silly). The dog is also blind and deaf, bumping into things. Where is the quality of life? What's our biggest fears. For her, we can at least consider choices. For me, she'll use up all of Dee's caregiver time and patience—leaving little for me.

But for me, now losing my senses, it feels like being buried alive.

I need a shrink to help me deal with whatever inconvenience and indignations I suffer, and THEN I die? Why is that my sentence? There are more than 7 billion people on earth. To what consequence is it if some want to be "excused" early? Don't I get a say in the matter?

So why do we euthanize our pets? To put an animal down is humane, right? Are we being humane? Why not be humane with humans? Landon laughed when the dog ran into a snow pile. Maybe it was funny like a blindfolded kid playing. Was Frankenstein funny? Will it come to a point when some ask, "does it now become a case of how much can I withstand or endure?" We treat our pets with more compassion! "They Shoot Horses, Don't They?"

Yet, I've been afforded the opportunity to breathe the air on this earth; why cut it short, regardless of its price? But, how much extra carbon dioxide is contributing to climate change simply because perhaps billions of more people are needlessly contributing to the atmosphere by extending their lives?

There are no do-overs, reruns, gimmes, or returns. Life's not a commodity available to all or on sale 24/7 forever or anytime. And maybe how they look at my end-days will be their problem to deal with. Why not breathe all the air that I can? So what, if I want an extra glass of wine or two; or three or four? I'm not that selfish or imposing. I got my "ticket" for this "ride" years ago. Now I'm not allowed to get off?

I have a shooting pain along with a dull and persistent pain in my eye. I also have been diagnosed with cataracts. Which is worse, having full-body neuropathy, or being blind and on withdrawal of steroids? Maybe one should be advised by their doctor? Maybe the doctor should read the medicines being taken in their questionnaires? Do they even read them?

From the Hospital for Special Surgery website:

> *"Steroids can sometimes cause cataracts or glaucoma or worsen these conditions if they are already present."*

From: Johns Hopkins Vasculitis Center:

> *"Prednisone is a corticosteroid. In contrast to anabolic steroids (used by "bodybuilders"), corticosteroids are used in inflammatory conditions for their anti–inflammatory effects."*

"

"They shut down the production of adrenaline produced by the Adrenal Gland and producing some of the side-effects which include: "Weight Gain; Glucose Intolerance; Hypertension; Increased Susceptibility to Infections; Bone Thinning; Easy Bruising; Mood Swings; Insomnia; Avascular Necrosis of bone; Abdominal Striae; Cataracts; Acne"

Check the side effects of your medicines and do your research! "It's not nice to fool Mother Nature." Prednisone, or steroids, are helpful, but they're also nasty drugs. They, and other drugs, can create symptoms unrelated to your illness. "Iatrogenic:" an illness or disease caused by medication or treatment. Also known as a reason to keep "chasing one's tail." A drug for this, and one for the side-effects of the drug?

* * *

One of my problems typing was that if my numbed fingers accidentally hit the "Cap Lock" key, without looking at the keyboard, I could be typing away in all capitals! Then I have to go back to the beginning of the caps and retype all that was capitalized, not knowing if there's a shorter method. So, I ripped the cap lock key off from the keyboard. The frustration motivated by Prednisone can sometimes serve some perverted purpose.

We had our family counselling session yesterday with in mind that I lived with my father's cancer every day for 10 years. I don't want to be grandpa to my own children. The important revelation from the session was that this affliction, my illness, affects everybody as a major life-changing event. Just like with my dad's cancer.

From the boys' recognition that their, once invincible, dad could possibly be diminished by some alien event, to Dee's acknowledgement that her husband was "taken away," only to be returned in some altered state, like *Invasion of the Body Snatchers*. They share in the feeling of alienness that my body is inflicting me with, and we kinda know what that looks like.

Sure, shit happens, but I say everyone would have been better off with my quicker death as opposed to the uncomfortable memories of some ongoing debilitating illness and slow disintegration of a once vibrant individual. That's like watching the pet cat slowly decompose—except I'm Dad!

Thinking back, I WAS grateful that my father survived about ten years after his diagnosis. But it came at a cost to him. Whether it was his medication or decrease in testosterone, he mellowed from the hard-ass that he was. And I was able to get to know him beyond my angry teen-years. The negative of his illness was transformed into a positive. But maybe my family would just like to keep me around. Be careful what you wish for.

If I'm being selfish because it'll all come at a cost, could living-on be my greatest expression of love for them regardless of my pain, discomfort, short-temperedness, and cost? Or is it my vanity that stands in the way of just experiencing all the facets of my life? Staying in my "man-cave" of a den is my elephant burial-ground.

* * *

I'm thinking of creating an ALS Ice bucket-styled challenge vs LGi1 neuropathy nerve regeneration? Bring it on!

The Centers for Disease Control and Prevention (CDC) estimate that between 14,500 and 15,000 people in the United States (U.S.) had ALS in 2016, with around 5,000 people receiving a diagnosis annually. Worldwide, it is thought to affect between 2 and 5 people in every 100,000.

We don't know the exact number of LGi1 Neuropathy suffers. From Medical News Today—

66 *"...Although the exact number of people with polyneuropathy is not known, the National Institute of Neurological Disorders and Stroke (NINDS) estimate that approximately 20 million people in the United States have some form of peripheral neuropathy, and most of them have polyneuropathy."* 99

I say, bring on that Ice Bucket Challenge! There's no reason you couldn't be next in experiencing this disease! For this, is just a roll of the dice. But response to, or treatment, shouldn't remain mysterious and unavailable. Too much medical and related expense goes into dealing with this illness not to address a solution that affects so many.

25

Anybody else feel the way I do?

August 20, a year after discharge. Now I like doing nothing. The tightness in the chest after eating, stressful situations, drinking wine, what's THAT all about? And it also seems to be getting, incrementally, worse each day, if that's real.

Maybe it's the heat?

We're in the Hamptons now for a couple of day's break, all alone, at a friend's house. Nice listening to the clear, blue tinted, water ripple in the pool while I do nothing. THAT'S a vacation! I have one thing that cooperates with me: my head. And that's, apparently, not 100% for now. But is that a reason to continue living with the rest of the misery? So, from the neck down, I have a mutiny on my hands. And from the shoulders up, it's questionable as to what bodily allegiances I CAN depend on.

The wife says I should just get used to it and let's move on. But until I have closure as to the ultimate prognosis, and that either something or nothing more can be done; then how do I get used to something that is so amorphous and inconclusive? Who wants to leave the "show" early?

I'll slowly be going into the sunset until that night ends as a Head-in-the-Bed. And planning for that event can't be too early. If I'm late then there's no one who can put me out of my, or our suffering.

I'm the one who has to ignore my symptoms for the benefit of others?

* * *

So far, even the lawyers won't touch my case because it's so complicated. But who made it complicated? I didn't start this health-clusterfuck by prescribing Augmentin. To understand what I'm going through, I tell others that I wish they could trade places with me for five minutes. Unfortunately, that's obviously impossible and doesn't really convey the feelings. So, I go through the motions of describing it again:

- I walk on feet wrapped around with cotton on duct tape and then shoved into shoes stuffed with tennis balls or socks.
- I feel like there are compression socks, on my legs, to the groin, and arms to the armpits.
- The hands are numb, prickly, and stiff. Sometimes they cramp.
- The trunk, or around my chest from the waist to the neck feels like there is a bullet-proof vest wrapped tightly around my chest.
- I move, and the muscles contract like in a spasm.
- It's difficult to turn my body to look over my shoulders.
- The autonomic issues of: blood pressure, fainting, gastro issues, sexuality, brain fog, fatigue, are too enumerable to repeat.

This is probably unbelievable or unfathomable to most. Are some bothered by how often I describe my ailment? Good! Now maybe with more of the repetition you'll get to experience, 1% of the time, what I, and other similar sufferers feel *all* of the time. This is not our imaginations!

* * *

I'm in an infusion center now, writing this in a reclining chair—just pondering my life. The Benadryl is starting to take effect.

Although there are other patients present, I still feel alone. I doubt anyone else has my affliction and symptoms. It may be comforting to compare notes and commiserate. But why bother? There's little to share. Others can't make me feel better. I don't get comfort from anyone else's misery.

At least these patients don't appear to walk like me. Of course, they have their issues, and never should any two cases be compared like this. All I can do, and along with the other people who come for treatment, is to endure, and trust that their doctors are on top of their game. But as we've seen played out here, don't bet the farm on it.

I try to live in my new world. I'm now attempting to read about interabled romance. Ben Matlin's, *In Sickness and in Health*. He was handicapped from birth. The story of a guy born with spinal muscular atrophy, "an incurable neuromuscular condition that has caused him to be quadriplegic," and a non-disabled, woman who married, had two children, and lived their lives happily ever after. But there's a difference. He was born with the disease. There was an attraction that began in that situation, and a mutually accepting desire to carve out a life together based on: "This is what we have."

For me, everybody's script as actors in a somewhat pedestrian family journey through life changed abruptly without any forewarning or choice...Now, new costumes for all! But at least I had the gift of good fortune to raise my family unencumbered with this challenging illness!

* * *

When Dee and I first met, we traveled to California that August for an end of summer road trip down the Pacific Coast Highway, Route 1, from SF to LA, stopping along the way to notable tourist attractions of Big Sur, the Hearst Castle, and Harmony, CA, just to name a few. I told her she was fun to travel with as we proceeded south on the outside of the roadway, with no guardrail. If I were any more nervous on the drive, for fear of heights, I could have easily gone over the edge.

While in the motel room one morning, Dee was greeted, as she came out of the shower, with a diamond engagement ring on the washing counter.

Yes, I had it in my pocket on the way out in the plane. Of course, she was shocked, said yes, and felt compelled to immediately tell the world. Which for her was, namely, her family.

But before we had all of these salivating family members on both coasts burning up the phone lines, I said, "Let's keep it our secret until we return." She did tell "Fred from Fresno" in the parking lot, though. A stranger satisfied her need to tell *someone*. But little could I foresee the road trip to come.

We were engaged three months after we met, and married within six, before she turned 27.

And noooo, it was not a shotgun wedding. I was just head over heels about her and felt the music had stopped for my dating. It was time to settle down and move on. Why delay? On such short notice we expected to have trouble finding a wedding site. It turned out that the upcoming Thanksgiving weekend was available where we wanted to be married. With that, we were off on a Honeymoon in Rio.

She was my pinup girl, better than any I thought I would meet from the pages of *Playboy*, or any other magazine for that matter. All unrealistically misleading the young stallions who thought the magazines were classifieds for "girls wanted." I think I realized that nobody's perfect (outside of me; ha!), and Dee would be the best thing to ever happen to me.

She had what I called "potential." Something unquantifiable that the person you know would have your back to the best of their ability and could be trusted to work with you, regardless of the hurdles to overcome. Turns out we agree on just about all the fundamentals. Except, whenever it comes to the kids, she's gate open: "Oh, it's all right." I'm gate closed; the disciplinarian.

Bryce simply recognized, we were/are Yin and Yang. Mars/Venus, maybe? Dee, being a nurse from a medical background primarily meeting clean-cut doctors, I was her fantasy guy with a big mustache and the hair to go with it. The cowboy without the disguise. But also, the guy with a temperament to match. I was Margaret Mitchell's Rhett Butler: "Frankly my dear…"

I know that sometimes I could be somewhat tough and disregarding feelings, particularly if, to me, the "principle" was more important than maintaining the peace. One can always make peace. It's taken me a long time to learn the opposite lesson. Particularly with the temperament-altering Prednisone, all bets are off. But for 34 years and counting, we've stuck through it all; over the mountains of euphoria, through the depths of yelling hell, and the plateaus of just living amidst the asparagus. Wouldn't trade my family package for anything. As they say, "In a sea of troubles, swim for your own." Unfortunately, now, the swim period is coming to a close and I feel like drowning.

I wonder where we'll go now. I'm slowly learning to live with my disability, and although realizing the end doesn't have to be near, the illness seems to stay ahead of me.

Along with cleaning toilets, Dee says she also won't cut my toenails. Cutting nails is a chore and a problem for me. And because I have difficulty bending, gripping, and manipulating a nail clipper, all the more difficult it is to perform the task, particularly with the shaking hands of a Parkinson's patient. I'm lucky if I don't draw blood. But where am I going? What's a drop of blood in my condition? Maybe I could cut my own toenails too short and bleed to death.

Every day is a new experience. What happens when things get worse? The family is loving. It makes me question: "What if the shoe was on the other foot?" How would I react if the tables were reversed? Would I look for ways out of the marriage or accept the cards as dealt and be as caring as Dee—until she's not?

There are perils to asking these questions. One may not like the answers. Like Mattlin says, "My disability becomes her disability." Maybe, also, in our case. But we weren't born like this and knowing beforehand what we were getting into. Although we can be in touch communicating multiple times a day, I can also give her some space; but the space is different. We used to be close sometimes. Now, it's not the same.

Now, we have little interaction other than a hug or a kiss. So, closing the gap is different. Probably for multiple reasons ranging from medications to autonomic issues, I barely have a libido aside from my heartbeat.

I still like the idea of sex. I still sneak a peek when she undresses, in the closet, and I yearn for something to stir. Oh, those boobs. But there's no connection between the brain and the rest of the gang. And there's little excitement attempting to arouse your partner while wearing the equivalent of oven-mitts over your hands. I'm so sorry.

* * *

Sunday morning, the day before Columbus Day, I'm supposed to start the urinary collection for a day and bring it over to Lab Corp. the next day for their analysis as per the instructions from the Hematologist. Lab Corporation being the acceptable, reimbursed testing facility for me. **Be sure your procedures are reimbursed. And ask, unless you like potential, surprise, unreimbursable, invoices.**

It occurred to me that maybe the place is closed on the "holiday" obviating the need for the sample. So, because the question popped into my mind, I posed it to Dee.

She rolls her eyes, makes a face, and I can see a fight brewing. Instead, I questioned her attitude, knowing that she thinks everything is about me. Well, right there that's a session for a head doctor which she should go to. She's tightly wound-up at this point.

Am I supposed to save these questions until I forget them? A simple answer could have been: "I don't know." But my brain now becomes obsessed with these concerns. Like an Alzheimer's sufferer, or Dustin Hoffman's *Rainman*, this is, now, who I am! Try telling them how their "script" should read. I simply expressed my disdain for her attitude, and accepted her difficulty with me and the issue. But she did apologize later on. Score one for Bob and one for the therapist. Being a "caregiver is not easy. The rug is constantly being pulled out from underneath.

So, I dropped the bomb of a question on my therapist. "Suppose the shoe were on the other foot?" Suppose I was healthy, and Dee was sick. Could I, would I, display the same empathy or caring as is displayed by some others? Or would I want a divorce?

I doubt the divorce; that's just changing one for a potential other, if someone would even have me at this point. But, I suppose, I might become detached. After all, wouldn't I have a business to run and a family to feed, sexual needs? Would I be justified as a product of my upbringing—male? Would it be selfish of me not to return the care? After all, it's what I learned from my mother caring for my father's cancer for 10 years, and sexually he was in the same position as I am. Weird, right? But what would the shoe on the other foot look like?

I learned, growing up, that if you have a fever you can stay out of work or school. Otherwise you went. Dee sometimes reminds me of a 13-year-old when she has a sore throat, without fever. Fortunately, that's been the extent of her illnesses. I have difficulty empathizing with her in that condition. It's really not a fair example, apples for apples. I have full body neuropathy and a bunch of other shit. She doesn't. But what it came down to was that I feel guilty about me blowing up everyone's lives. Maybe part of ending my life is the termination of my guilt. My gal therapist says: "While you're here, get what you can."

So, I asked her what's the consensus on this as to where billions of people end up? Do they express the same concerns or issues as I? She said, "There's no clear-cut path. We all have to experience it ourselves." So I said, "That's good for another 6-12 months of therapy."

I wanted to know what the human universals are that would give us that consensus as to where we would most likely end up? Billions of people have experienced similar feelings through their human universals. How have they dealt with it? What did they discover? Why are we reinventing the wheel? Just because we're individuals in thought, doesn't mean we're individuals in existence. We're part of a herd.

* * *

Are you going to tell me that I would have to endure my torture just so an insurance company could say I died of natural causes so that they wouldn't question the payout if I was compelled to end my life because of some depressive state caused by this illness? This torture is what would make me want to die because it would be natural to want to end my misery! No? Who, in their right mind, can live like this? At least, why don't we get termination by choice? If I'm the one living in this condition, I, alone, should have the right to end it!

I talked to my shrink about hope, which in my pragmatist's terminology is potential. Dr. Hematologist's opinion was that nerve regeneration can take up to a decade or more. Then there really is little potential at this time. My life expectancy is only less than ten years, anyway, so what's the point? Where's the "potential" when the clock runs out? When there is little potential for recovery and my future is living in my mobile torture cell, then despair sets in with little to look forward to. Just more of the same deteriorating, exhausting days.

The price to pay for less potential becomes more of a risk/reward analysis. What's the payoff compared to my investment of the cost of the torture?! And I'm hardly alone.

It's not like I'm thirty years old and I have my whole life before me with kids, energy, and all, and this is one of life's "cards" I've been dealt. Then, there's far more to consider.

But at this point, I'm just trying to be practical, and not falsely optimistic. Some may say practicality shouldn't enter the discussion when it comes to living a life. I say, again: "when do you want to stand in my shoes, and then tell me what price you'd pay not to trade back with me so you wouldn't be chasing your tail?" Are we living in the real world or a Utopia?

Sorry. But as you can see, I'm not capable of performing on a healthy person's level. I'm confronting my unconventional mortality, you're not. My job was done, and before I leave I don't have to make sure I make the bed for you!

Making an appointment six months out is pretty optimistic on the part of the Hematologist, particularly when my affliction is still advancing. If there's little the doctors can do, what's the point of the follow-up visit? Establishing an annuity for others? I'm not making contributions.

What kind of vegetable will I be in six months? And then, what's my vegetable half-life? How will this vegetable-to-be present itself? More cooked than now, or in the same state, raw? Maybe Dee doesn't see or understand the gravity of the situation. I will not be a Head-in-the-Bed. I don't want to be an over-roasted, picked-at, pickled-cauliflower revenue stream either!

I've spent the past year waiting within the system, enduring the unabated creeping progression of this illness, while the medical community remains baffled, all to no avail. It's not even punting. The IVIGs and a couple of pills are really all that's been tried over the last year, and for naught. Meanwhile, I vacillate between not giving in to all the temptations, and acquiescing to the weight of the transformation.

I'm not asking my family for approval or consent; rather more for understanding, love, and support for my choices to end this life that I, now, must call, mine.

Who's really the selfish ones here? How dare the naysayers sentence me to an endless, unyielding torture chamber.

Because simply it wouldn't be politically or religiously correct to advocate such a position? I said it was sad that what's before me is my future. An abrupt end for my life as envisioned. "Sure Bob, go do yourself in." I'm not alone in my situation. Regardless that many others have different circumstances, it doesn't mean they're not feeling tormented, or they simply suffer from depression to be marginalized, discounted, and relegated to the trash-bin: untreatable.

> *"There comes a time, thief, when the jewels cease to sparkle, when the gold loses its luster, when the throne room becomes a prison, and all that is left is a father's love for his child."*

--John Milius, Conan's King Osric

26

Reality Check

Now that Bryce has made it clear that he frowns on my delving into another restaurant location, because he believes we have enough debt which will impede retirement. I can only guess that things in my life are going to get totally boring.

Maybe being bodysnatched isn't such a bad thing at all? What, with selling stocks, no new restaurant, less doctor's appointments, all I can likely look forward to are the occasional infusions. I won't have as many "toys" to keep me occupied or get me into trouble.

I mean, how many times can I refresh the NY Times webpage or any other page for that matter? How many times can I refresh the catering order page, waiting for a new order to come in, knowing full well that orders only come in once a week! And if I'm not busy with something, I can certainly find a way to get into trouble. Maybe a life living in a psych ward after a lobotomy might be just what the doctors should order for me. But that costs taxpayers and the family, too.

Yesterday was an ugly day. Bryce, my oldest came for a visit but I think there was more of an agenda on his part. After his chatting with Dee for a while, he comes into my space and eventually it builds into a shouting match that I shouldn't bully his mom. He did this, of course, without inquiring as to why she felt bullied or my interpretation of the situation. Next thing you know, Landon and Jesse are also in the room and I'm the target. Unfortunately, since I'm on Prednisone, to me, all bets are off when it comes to my owning the behavior to the fullest degree. Prednisone is responsible for "memory loss, paranoia, sadness, and many psychotic tendencies," so reported by Google. The internet is loaded with testimonials to this effect. So, I'm not making this stuff up or as an excuse. I can't discount its intrusion into my behavior. Nor should anyone else.

But it was a Saturday Night Massacre and a buildup of more than a year's worth of elephant shit in the room. But we did end the evening just short of doing the Kumbaya. The last thing I want is to go to bed "unfriending" my kids.

The ugly memories that I have will be endured and dealt with for a far shorter time than the others who are younger who also share similar memories. Make the best out of what's remaining of your time with me. Shitty memories with recriminations have a way of surviving. Shakespeare's, Mark Antony speaking about the death of Caesar: "The evil that men do lives after them; the good is oft interred with their bones." Sixth grade was memorable for something.

Is Dee so steady or stable a person that her endurance with my shit over the last 18 months hasn't affected her? What does she hear when complaining of what I've said? How does she hear it? Does she think I'm demeaning her, criticizing her complaint? That's the farthest thing from the truth. Why would I do that and jeopardize the hand that helps care for me? And make sure you have the right enemy. Maybe she, also, needs therapy? Or will death be my only way out for her? Is "'till death do us part" an unreasonable oath? Or do we trust it'll evolve?

* * *

Bryce checked in with a recap of last week's Saturday night massacre. We both felt badly that it occurred, but he reminded me that we're all a family finding our way through this mess and not to worry. We're a family in love, far different than the family I grew up in. Dee's influence of course. But I've caught on.

And if love is the base for the building, we sometimes can do alterations in progress for the family unit. I asked if I would be having a test on what he was telling me to emphasize that he was talking a lot. Fortunately, he said, "no." I know I'm slowing down. But he's beyond me. Although he did mention that he did notice another side of me when he reflected on Saturday's episode. He said, "now he knows where he got 'it' from."

I'm very lucky to have these three boys for my sons. If I could have picked them from a store window I couldn't have selected better. If I were walking in the snow and the boys were behind me, I think they would be close to, if not in my footsteps.

I think they get it; far better than I. Dee and I have done a good job. What more could I learn from them but what they have filled their own minds with? But if I want to know what they've learned, it'll come at a cost; and a greater one than if I were healthy. Do all parents have to learn what their children have learned to appreciate their accomplishments?

We trust all children exceed their parent's knowledge and position by having been exposed to opportunity and given space to explore. Progress is not walking for 40 years in the same footsteps down that mine shaft as your father walked. Kids have their own minds to explore. And if they don't, then we as parents haven't done our jobs, and may have possibly failed.

My father and mother never said, "I Love you." to each other or even to me, that I can recall. Never the hugs or even an arm-around. No touching. I guess I was sensory deprived. Or let's put it this way, it wasn't said enough that I believed it or remembered from that authoritarian era.

But years ago, I saw a father and son hug and kiss on the cheek and thought it was a nice expression of their love for each other; without anyone sitting on some jury. Men didn't kiss or hug in my father's world. As a child I was not raised as such. But apparently, I took note. "How ya going to keep them down on the farm after they've seen Paris?"

I feel like the character Wikus van der Merwe from the 2009 Peter Jackson film, *District 9.* The protagonist of that science fiction story slowly undergoes a physical metamorphosis from human to insectile alien. Starting with facial discoloration and growths to the body, to an eventual complete transformation into an alien species. Seems like I'm not far behind.

I know; how many lobsters have I killed and eaten in my lifetime? Plenty. This metamorphosis is payback time from the lobster gods. Thinking about it, I crawl across the floor like one, my chest feels like that body armor wrapped around the midsection of Mr. Lobster, and my hands now operate like those two weird things for claws; that they can only pinch and feel something between the two hammers or pincers. They couldn't feel the edges of their clothes like I can't with my fingers. They certainly couldn't feel but they could pinch. I can't even do that now! But sitting high above their body sits their eyes and antenna while whatever brain they possess directs all their traffic of movements to their extremities—just like mine! I AM turning into an insect or a lobster!

* * *

I can't imagine what could come from the Dec. 10, NYU meeting. How could they possibly tell me something new that would lead me to continue unless they see something all the others haven't? Otherwise, they're just another baffled or handcuffed facility observing my helpless condition. And frankly, what am I doing taking all of this IVIG treatment some $20,000 per dose? If the government can subsidize farmers not to grow crops, thereby maintaining a higher price, why not subsidize wheelchair shlunkers to save money and misery. Use the savings from decreased medical expenses for human growth. Aren't there hungry and deserving kids who could benefit more from a swap or redirection of funds? You can have mine. Instead of paying $20k for my, useless, 'till end-of-life treatments, give the patient a settlement of say, $10k for each in exchange for no more medical care, and save the rest to the system! Give the savings to more deserving medical or social care for the more vibrantly surviving or growing.

* * *

From: QJM: An International Journal of Medicine, Oct 2012

Why trunc*al neuropathy should be recognized:*

" *"...Our cases illustrate the consequences of unrecognized truncal neuropathy to the clinician and patient. For the clinician, the unexplained pain poses a diagnostic challenge and investigation for differential diagnoses is sought. Unfortunately, these investigations are unrewarding.*

The patient who is already troubled by pain is asked to undergo a range of different investigations, requiring multiple hospital visits, contributing to anxiety. Furthermore, treatment with effective analgesia is delayed in the continued hope of establishing a diagnosis.

"

Early recognition of truncal neuropathy avoids unnecessary investigation, minimizes patient anxiety and allows prompt-effective pain management. ..."

And that shouldn't be limited to the mysteries of Neuropathy. I'm not the only patient with a difficult-to-diagnose ailment. When are a patient's reasonable expectations unreasonable, or worthy of an independent review committee in these extraordinary cases? What we're really doing, as patients with weird illnesses, is permitting Doctors to practice on us without guidance or supervision against over-eager doctors from saying they are simply treating a rare case for cover from scrutinization. When is "millions of patients" rare? Guarding their pride and egos by hiding behind laws permitting, in essence, experimentation under the guise of "treatment," without any consequences? Perhaps there should be a central reviewing committee hearing about these strange cases and immediately move them to a more responsible or capable jurisdiction. Maybe we should be heading to some centralized medical care for cost savings if not expediency to solving cases. So, why do we limit lawsuit damages to some degree because the system doesn't recognize there could be an alternate, more efficient solution?

The crime here is that a doctor's ignorance, ego or pride, possibly, came between me and the answer as to treatment. Because he was a duck out of water or unfamiliar with the situation, he didn't, a) ask someone else for help, b) ask someone else for help soon enough, or c) ask someone else for help. Dickweed!

Our health system needs to be centralized with a database to prevent cases like mine and others from losing time and duplicating unnecessary and costly treatment. A database with a red flag, and a little Artificial Intelligence, in the master chart, would have shown an alarm to the potential limit of Augmentin dosage. If you've administered the wrong drugs, the red flag goes up and says, "You're in the process of fucking up the patient; undo, undo."

HIPAA will just have to be modified a little. I mean, old people gab more about their illnesses than any doctor can give away any secrets to another. Just make sure the patient's info isn't sold to outsiders like insurance companies. Besides, who cares about the likes of some ole' lady's hemorrhoids? Can you imagine the unnecessary expense being absorbed by the health system overlapping treatment because every doctor gets their own whack at the problem? How about, professionally, rating doctors with regard to success rate, field, and some other important characteristics, and parcel out the "difficult" cases to the more intelligent and capable doctors?

From John Hopkins Medicine:

> "*Nerve damage in neuropathy progresses sooner than previously thought, lending urgency to earlier detection and treatment.*"

> "*... early neuropathy tends to progress,*" *says Michael Polydefkis '93, a professor of neurology and the paper's senior author. "Primary care doctors should always take it seriously, even if the patient is just talking about slight numbness.*"

Why does health come down to who gets the best care? Why don't all patients receive care that makes the most sense instead of the luck of the draw when it comes to who's giving the care? I used to believe that in many cases, an accused criminal is as guilty or innocent as their lawyer is effective. How about doctors?

One would think that with today's day and age of communication there are bulletins issued throughout the medical community alerting them to the possibility of pending issues and potential repercussions.

Why does it come down to who went to some convention to hear about something new and important? Having been to a few conventions, I know I haven't seen or heard it all. Why do we believe doctors are different? Architects receive updated building codes on a regular basis. Our automobiles get recalled. Heck, it seems to me that a disease as horrific and widespread as neuropathy and neurologically related illnesses deserve a simple bulletin so medical practitioners can file just such a note of possibility in the back of their minds. If you're missing a diagnosis or early warning sign that affects some 10% of the US population, I would say how much could issuing a bulletin cost vs. the ongoing expense of detecting and the almost futility of treating neuropathy? A conflict of interest, perhaps? Or is the neurological horizon of study one of those frontiers that doctors find they can comfortably, and discretely, wander about for the rest of their careers? Which neurologist says: "I got this."

Or is it really a matter of increasing the population of giving-cows acting as an annuity for the medical profession? Why should they be motivated to "solve the case" and end revenues when the American healthcare system is based on profit? Bill more, make more. Unheard of—out of the question?

From Harvard Medical School Harvard Health publishing:

> "Once you treat the underlying cause, does the neuropathy go away?" "Yes, if you treat it early and your nerve fibers are otherwise healthy," Dr. Oaklander says.

"The peripheral nerves keep growing throughout life. Just like broken bones, nerves will heal and regrow if you can remove the source of injury and protect them while they heal."

Why aren't we recognizing and treating this illness earlier?

Well, apparently no one diagnosed my condition early enough? And if they did, what did they do? Or is poo continued to be thrown against the wall because, in the meantime, it pays some bills. Unfortunately, although we still don't know the cause of my neuropathy except that it's idiopathic, autoimmune related (sounds like another cop-out), I could have been given an aggressive "anti-Neuropathy treatment." Except now, sounds like no nerve regeneration (if, at all) if we haven't removed the source. But maybe they didn't react soon enough. Even NYU said if early enough maybe something could have been done. But maybe, few know what to do because they've been to too many conventions. "Just sayn'." Or maybe just be straight with the patient. The science hasn't caught up to the illness.

Seems like that dog kennel sent me to Mt. Saini only because they're affiliated with them. But maybe they just hitched their wagon to any "star" for economic (for-profit) reasons. And maybe I should have been transported to another facility that specializes in my situation. Come to think of it, I was in the wrong hospital.

How many others are in the same situation without realizing it. Who says that someone received the best treatment just because they got out of a hospital in a somewhat stabilized condition? Does leaving the hospital with a limb cut off signify that they got the best treatment? Or could another facility have saved the limb altogether? You can't tell me two auto-body repair shops do the exact same job.

But maybe a paying patient in-hand is worth something more to them than the motivation to giving the right care, if they even can. With the variability of today's mores, are all doctors more interested in care vs. profit? Mt. Saini is a well-known liver transplant institution affiliated with the NJ institution but, as far as I know, hardly known for their neurological expertise. Although they may not have known at the time because of my spaghetti-bowl-like presentation; when they cleaned it up and isolated some clear-cut symptoms, perhaps they should have known they were in over their heads and transported me to a more tuned-in facility.

27

Am I the Big Fish?

So, while I now pass my days with an afternoon movie; I like love or romance stories. I like daddy stories. I like dying stories. It may all be related that I see, sentimentally, the end in sight.

I was touched by the movie, *Big fish.* The story of a son who has only heard tales about his father and believes they are nothing but tales—the son doesn't "know" his dad.

So, the story reviews his dad's life, and because of the way things were interpreted, by the end, the dad's life was revealed. I was touched by the tale, and as I lay for my two-hour morning meditation rise; I too reviewed my life.

It started with questions to a fortune teller, as lots of teens do: "Will I be rich?" To which the reply: "No, but you'll receive little gifts." So, some 60 years later I too, as others, have a story to tell for my life. And all things considered, my little gifts have made me wildly enriched. My books, a restaurant feeding thousands, and the family, building houses-to-be-homes, cooked charity meals for many, and it's travels through life adding to the narrative.

I think back on the things I've done and how their outcomes became gifts of a sort. Like the time I was about eight-years old and played Cowboys and Indians with my neighbor-friend, with real steel-tipped arrows. Accidents can happen while playing. And as I play-threatened my neighbor, the little Indian, pointing the arrow at his head, the arrow discharged and bounced off his bony eyebrow—not a quarter inch below deflecting into his eye socket. The gift was the story. Not as told, but what was avoided; as it could have been a disaster for all. Fortunately, the only damage done was his mom's "going through the roof" at me. For me, maybe it wasn't one of my best 8-year-old's ideas.

So, the elephant in my room has been confronted. As the therapist says, it's underneath what aggravates or accentuates the other issues. Through a few therapy sessions in my life, I've learned our emotions have a life of their own. They're like a balloon that's being squeezed—the bumps come out in different places. But they're still there.

My deep question to my gal therapist centered on the fact that I feel badly for Dee. I control her future. It's like I'm in prison for life and she's in the visiting room always waiting for me. Or like I'm taking her down a tunnel that's closed at the end. Where's her freedom, her control, her say in her predicament? She's trapped! The solution for Dee is my termination. It frees her up.

Did caregivers sign off to this contract? Nooo. Before one signs a contract they're entitled to know all the conditions before signing. Was my condition of what would come 35 years later, evident on our wedding day? Sure, we're in love. But is that love categorical regardless that the subjects are essentially different, in 35 years? "Till death do us part?" That's like buying a potential Super-fund cleanup site. Or getting a Jack-in-the-box for a wedding present and told to wait 35 years before opening.

I remember my mother taking on my father, with his prostate cancer, as a contracted wedding vow, "whither thou goist," and then 40 years later him complaining that she's bullying him because illness makes us frail and vulnerable. I remember my mother-in-law tending to her husband who had Parkinson's. Unfortunately, she predeceased him from breast cancer. Did she miss a beat while loving him? Just shit happens?

I get Dee's disappointment, sadness, denial and depression. It's a no-win situation for her, as it was for her mother. That just makes three of us. Now what? What are the choices? Who pays? The luck of the draw for a situation that we will all confront? With our "great" advancements in medical care—we've not considered all the repercussions.

Now, my exercise therapy appointments, my eye checkups, my NYU doctor appointments, and all the other issues that concern me are moved to the top of *her* to-do lists? Unless she declares; "I'm all yours." The overlaying little jobs of taking out the garbage, tending the dog, the kids, the store, life—now supersede her life just because I got hit first by a truck?

Am I keeping her against her will or do we live with the simmering pot under the sheets? I'm responsible. Only, I have a key to set her free?

Why do I make it about sex? Or is that more of a guy thing? All I know is that Dee said today that she appreciated the acknowledgement of my feelings toward her. I guess she was feeling the same way; that I was controlling her destiny without much of a choice for her. She commented that we'll find a way and that the boys felt tuned into our plight. I was relieved to hear her words of support and commitment. I guess she'd rather spend a life with me, disability and all, without sex, than no life at all. But that may just be a fantasy.

I think, as a guy, I may have some priorities mixed up.

So, why does it come down to sex in my thoughts when it's more than a year and a half since anyway?

And how would I respond if the shoe was on the other foot; if Dee was the afflicted one and I was healthy? But wait. It's plenty complicated trying to answer the first set of questions and issues. Who needs further mentally masturbated complications?

Now, I'm making resolutions and shedding the weight of the issues I've been carrying around that have only complicated things. I've given up the idea of a new location for the store because it's not only about me. I'm a new man, resigned and accepting of my physical restrictions and condition. Even though the NYU Dysautonomia Center sent me home with a prescription for a sleep test and with a blood pressure monitor. It's little other than more chazerai (or junk) as they say. Each new doctor gives hope like they're some newfound Messiah. But the "pro" of hope can't last forever. And disappointment with the ultimate conclusion is often the result.

* * *

I sit here with a sigh while contemplating my condition. My feet up on an ottoman to limit the swelling. My belly feeling as if a large medicine ball was sitting on my stomach.

I'm tired of dragging this illness around. The hands and fingers work so poorly that when I blow my nose and wipe it, and when inspecting the tissue, as guys would do, surprise, finger through the tissue! I'm becoming stiffer when I have to turn my body when driving or even getting out of the car. The torso is tighter around my belly, shoulders, and arms, up to the neck.

But if I continue deteriorating like this, I suppose I would be described as being the most courageous, and the most exceptional role model. "We are the Heroes" as Queen would say. And probably the biggest gluttons for punishment in the pursuit of clinging to our one gift, the gift to experience life. How I was seen really would come down to being a coward if I ended my life regardless of the discomfort, difficulty, and pain. And probably I'd be rationalizing it all and just making the best out of a bad situation if I didn't. But you know what? I'm the only one living in my body.

Who knows how I'll be doing in a few months' time? Did I live on with whatever remains of my life? Did I succumb to the weight of this illness, or do I continue to suck out every last agonizing breath while torturing everyone else with my pains and needs? My gal therapist said: "Take what you can." I know there has to be equilibrium somewhere—not simply waiting 'till death—game over.

So, the transformation is almost complete, but to what? I don't know how this ends, but I also don't know my durability or endurance. I pay a price every day. The question is, do I see a trade off?

No more the fond memories of the boys riding the imaginary motorcycle on dad's knees, or my swinging them around my shoulders onto my back and asking: "Where's Daddy?" Where *is* Daddy? Those times are, now, light-years passed.

I watched *Mandalorian* tonight. That along with Twinkies and Yankee Doodles, or Yodels, could keep me interested in life a little longer. And of course, the last episode of the Star Wars trilogy comes out in about two weeks. Can't miss that with my boys. But thinking about it, in my lifetime, I've seen every episode of Star Wars and four modern presidential impeachments, all real-time. Those numbers of people, who can claim the same, are probably few and far between. But "thanks Medicare," for enabling the frivolous spending on extending the end of my tortured life.

* * *

Meanwhile, I had a decent dinner with Dee and Landon. We broached the subject of suicide, where I actually heard from Dee that she said she would support taking my own life if that's what I wanted, and maybe she would assist with a method. Now we're talking. Or maybe that's Dee's short-answer solution to last week's nearly pre-divorce argument—just "yes" me. We're talking cluster-fuck here mixing all that's at hand. Landon also didn't want to stand in my way as though he understood my needs. I believe his being a psych major in college, knowing who his dad is, helps him with some compassion in this situation. But here comes the disrupter. Dee and I met with the NYU group at the Dysautonomia Center...

28

A New Sheriff's in Town

And he has a posse. A team, really, of international doctors who are interested in the, just about, complete rarity of my illness, confirming that I seem to be one-of-a-kind. In other words, I'm royalty, of a pure lineage, one-of-a-kind for someone in my condition with the combination of my symptoms.

Just when one thinks they're at wits' end, along comes someone to turn over the cart; the cheugy, old way of thinking, and offers a new perspective. Let's just bark up another tree. The giving cow is sucked into the diagnostic vortex, once again, that tunnel of possibilities and non-directional, hope.

I got some straight talk, and I also received some new talk which now has to be digested on everybody's part. Because we're dealing with what few have heard about. This revised journey we're all about to embark on will force us to think and operate from a new perspective," outside of the box." Because, if I gain little from this expedition, at least there'll be some contributing study (on me) offering some guidance for future potential sufferers.

As a practical matter, I would say that if there are so few patients available in my condition, then why waste the money and maybe that's why drug companies don't bother with small-market drugs. But I'm thinking like a researcher who's thinking on a day/rate basis: "What have we learned today?" But they don't think about the short term. What's gleaned today is a building block for the future. That I understand. The chase—like dating for the capture, is sometimes the challenge—even if it doesn't end as desired or planned. A consolation prize in this respect is the possible discovery as aid to the unknown future sufferers. Maybe it's giveback time. Maybe I can get some part of the grant too? Seems only fair. Even a prisoner gets a day's pay for prison work.

Although, I think I've been rather emphatic that I wasn't going to be a guinea pig. But that wasn't considering some new light on the issues and perhaps a different viewpoint.

After performing a critical Tilt-Table Test, the new NYU team, from the Dysautonomia Center, has a suspicion that my illness could be Autoimmune Autonomic Neuropathy, or in the vicinity of Ganglionopathy; which would explain the lack of Encephalitis. But also include, according to NIH's National Center for Advancing Translational Sciences:

"What causes autoimmune autonomic ganglionopathy?

The cause of autoimmune autonomic ganglionopathy is not fully understood.[1] An autoimmune component is presumed, as the body's own immune system damages a receptor in the autonomic ganglia (part of the peripheral autonomic nerve fiber)... About 60% of cases follow an infection or other illness."

Maybe like the stubborn chest virus in my case? The late doubletalking, Professor Irwin Corey couldn't have explained it better.

"Some people with autoimmune autonomic ganglionopathy present with POTS-like symptoms."

Sounds like me! And because of the combination and permutation of the variable number of symptoms, my combination and extent, can render all of us, almost each as one-of-a-kind.

From The Cleveland Clinic website:

"Postural Orthostatic Tachycardia Syndrome (POTS) is a condition that affects circulation (blood flow). It involves the autonomic nervous system (which automatically controls and regulates vital bodily functions) and sympathetic nervous system (which activates the fight or flight response)..."

"Among the most common are: Neuropathic POTS: Peripheral denervation (loss of nerve supply) leads to poor blood vessel muscles, especially in the legs and core body..."

"...In summary, our study showed that POTS patients have deficits in specific areas of cognitive function including selective attention, processing speed, and executive function."

From: Vanderbilt Autonomic Dysfunction Center. Amy Arnold, PhD:

"...One of the most common symptoms reported by POTS patients is cognitive dysfunction or 'brain fog.' These terms both indicate a loss of brain functioning in areas such as thinking, remembering, concentrating, and reasoning to a level that interferes with daily activities.

> *In our center (Vanderbilt University's Autonomic Dysfunction Clinic), approximately 80 to 90% of POTS patients report cognitive dysfunction and often describe it as: "difficulty thinking, concentrating, or paying attention; trouble remembering things; cloudy or fuzzy feeling in head; and having problems finding the right words..."*

That's me! That's what I call my beffuddledness. You can't see these symptoms but you risk being called a "ditz brain," or some other uncomplimentary adjectives because it's difficult to empathize with the invisible.

The main problem is: the available science hasn't afforded the community the ability to prescribe a drug as a preventative or cure. And although there are millions of sufferers, according to Dysautonomia International, with some form of this illness, 70 million voices haven't been heard and targeted for a cure. We are the "kitchen junk drawer" of medical ailments. But when a series of similar symptoms are noted on a data base, a Tilt-Table Test should be mandated to confirm this widespread illness rather than continuing to chase our tails in a vacuum of knowledgeable professionals.

From their website:

> *"Dysautonomia is an umbrella term used to describe several different medical conditions that cause a malfunction of the Autonomic Nervous System.*

The Autonomic Nervous System controls the "automatic" functions of the body that we do not consciously think about, such as heart rate, blood pressure, digestion, dilation and constriction of the pupils of the eye, kidney function, and temperature control. People living with various forms of dysautonomia have trouble regulating these systems, which can result in lightheadedness, fainting, unstable blood pressure, abnormal heart rates, malnutrition, and in severe cases, death."

If the symptoms show up en mass—certainly, do the test immediately!

The new theory for my issue is that the dysfunction of, and all my symptoms of the autonomic system, is a result of the neuropathy. Autoimmune Autonomic Nervous system (AAN) and the autonomic system isn't really one system, but a group of individual components. But what set off the neuropathy or is it just a concurrent symptom of something else? And what's with the LGi1? Since I don't have encephalitis, the puzzle remains incomplete. But Mayo did the same test. Why wasn't our Wizard, back then, guided accordingly?

Did I hear that maybe my Myelin sheathing and nerves weren't fried? IF the NYU team is correct, then I could possibly have a diagnosis. And then, perhaps, a treatment could be offered; or, at least, have a clue that we're lost in the AAN wilderness?

A lot of ifs. Too many to make any sense that could be real or meaningful.

29

A change of heart? Grasping at straws?

Now I'm thinking about acupuncture, and or meditation, or even yoga. Others even mentioned salts, mechanics, and some other esoteric things. Apparently Western medicine can't even decide on a diagnosis or let alone, a cause for what I have. So, what have I got to lose trying to treat my symptoms of discomfort? A few bucks to indulge those with their recommendations? The skeptic that I am may be doubtful as to a simple cure or some relief that may come of these techniques. But it is silly not to try as a last-ditch effort. Yes, No, maybe?

I started this unwanted journey of discovery believing I couldn't endure and only wished for a, maybe self-interested, end to my life. When in actuality, I've lasted 586 days since entering the hospital. And next week is vacation.

So, maybe those in my position should be given some slack for a different outlook. Something to get used to. Maybe I'm a *Men in Black* where I can secretly tilt some part of the world's view to a different perspective. We can write the story anyway we want. But don't prejudge or make blanket statements that everyone falls under one category and therefore we can't, individually and with integrity, maintain some ultimate destiny and control over our lives, including the end to our lives. Talk about government or religious intrusion into making personal decisions. I'm not talking about a Jim Jones, Jamestown-type, drink-the-Koolaid mind-fuck here. I'm talking about making the decision to control the circumstances concerning the logical and acceptable end of my life.

They make you have babies against your will, make you pay extraordinary amounts for healthcare, if you can even get it, and tell some to go off to war. Then with all the misery, and more, you're told to endure it for the rest of your natural life. Isn't that cruel and unusual punishment, and because of the luck of the draw?! We treat our pets with more consideration!

As of now eleven states have an "End of Life" or "Death with Dignity" option. The problem with those options is: the patient must be terminally ill and death has to appear imminent within 6 months. Now we know why they're revered as "God"-like; "predictors of death." Who else would be bestowed with the ability to foretell life expectancy? Well, usually cancer-type patients who will die as a direct result of the illness can avail themselves of this option. But what about those incarcerated with their own bodily torture-cells without a cure? Those who feel their lives have been sent to some French penal colony. That's a double-edged sword. You get to stay on the Earth but with your hands and feet tied behind your back, stranded on some island with boiling frogs, or worse! I feel like saying the Greek's expression: "Skata!"

But maybe it's not just us and the question of if we can bear it. There's a whole larger ecosystem here that involves more than just us alone with our feelings. I may elect not to run to the next doctor's visit, knowing there's little reward in doing so. But I can be around to experience whatever comes from my wife, kids, and who knows what can follow. I am very fortunate, regardless of whatever shit I stepped into, and I don't want to take that from anybody if they so insist. And then maybe others can also see the light as to what other people in my condition experience.

Now, how much ya love me?

30

Rebooting the rest of my life

What *can* I do?

When my mind and body permit, I abound with creative energy; recipes and ideas for my restaurant; thoughts about social injustice and inequality, organization; too many things that still interest me and that I would like to do or investigate, wishful thinking for my kids to dream and think about.

It would be a shame to just shove all of my humanness into some crematorium, to be, almost instantly, incinerated and vanished forever. It's like throwing out all the boxes from grandma's attic into a dumpster, without ever even checking the contents. Once the hard drive is disposed of, that's the end. But maybe, to others, there's little interest in my thoughts, or value in my contributions. I mean, if the populous has become amenable to the likes of science deniers and inhumaneness to humanity, then what's the point of my fighting to be heard, when the populous, apparently, couldn't care less? At least, my kids are equipped to find their own path.

I can continue to oversee the restaurant. Maybe redirect our energy to updating and adding to the menu and increase sales after returning from this year's winter vacation. All with the goal of selling the business.

I can also explore a different tact to my health. I can pursue Eastern medicine which involves a more holistic approach of acupuncture, acupressure, meditation, CBD, and whatever else avails to a try. Those methods, of course, if the NYU team meets a dead end. But as of now, unless some miracle occurs, I don't think this is really a story that contains a happy ending. There are no miracles. Robin Williams was there before me. This one I could be heading straight to the trash bin. The professionals frozen with the inability to cure or prevent the illness.

And, yet I still like to write about this whole adventure for insight, as frustrating as it may be. But, for now, other than the typing difficulty and the physical imprisonment, my brain is still working.

Nothing can take it away. Nothing can take all of the difficulties experienced with this illness away from my body. No one can stop my brain. But at this point, I am living an exceptional life. And nothing should be scary, except Hamlet's incertitude.

How does one throw it away, and at what cost? The end is so finite!

* * *

I'm sitting outside on a terrace high above the Pacific Ocean on the Costa Rican coast. The mind still races ahead, the body lags far behind.

I feel like I'm waiting for something.

For what though? If I get out, what will I miss? Another volcano; another monkey jungle; all the feeble, remakes and reruns of 30-year-old movies? All the old oohs and aws to be put back until next time? There's little new under the sun, to paraphrase Shakespeare. It's all been reruns and reorganizations of old ideas and materials. We haven't brought any new things back from the beyond.

The other day I spent 45 minutes with three remotes trying just to put on a TV with sound. I could have assembled a 747 airliner with more ease. I look for the shortest way, weaving between the furniture to get to the other side. Everything's a chore or a challenge. I'm in beautiful Costa Rica inside watching the mindless movie, Armageddon.

I'm ok for now. But missing what I would do in the past and not wanting to burden or hold others back is what concerns me. I'm passing backwards past milestones of ability. Can I predict what my next loss will be?

Dunno.

Sometimes I just stand up and remain motionless like our old dog, Savanna, when she stands there staring at the air. We have that in common. And in that, I'm not alone. If I could disappear into the landscape, it would suit me just fine. Without a trace, just like when a child asks: "Where do all dead birds go?" Savanna's going to the same place, and she doesn't even care about writing a book. And the Christmas carols and inane Easter bunnies will continue, unabated, for many to be blithely happy. I want to go where the dead birds go. I like Savanna's recipe for "the end."

Maybe it is time to check out. With all the latest gadgets my kids play with and not having grown up with them, I feel like I'm on the outside of the box. I vacillate back and forth, wanting to endure and be here, or depending on the discomfort, not. We're all Hamlets. We think too much. Zippers are a nightmare. Jackets with zippers and pockets are still ferocious opponents. That should be our biggest concern. Meanwhile, at my age, there's always a Larry David moment. Always perks being handicapped and traveling. Always a zipper to be pissed at.

Had another spat with Dee. She complained that she wasn't asking for having to serve some of my needs. I said I didn't ask for this illness any more than she asked for giving more attention and care to her husband than she expected. So now we have a conundrum.

Now, how much ya love me?

* * *

Who wants to get dressed when you're warm and cozy, waking from a night's sleep without any urgency in getting out of the house? So, what, I'm in my pj's all day? Who wants to get all wet taking a shower? Shaving? Brushing teeth? Like, helloooooo, those daily obsessive compulsive behaviors are only promulgated by the neurotics governed by a 24-hour clock. My clock is governed by hygienics, not hours...

But we're in a Covid world now. The behavior required to outlast something that's both new and that has been around for eons is now forcing us to adapt our 24-hour clocks to something else. I, for one, am now essentially quarantined. Which means I don't interact with the outside world's timetable. It doesn't matter when I wake, shower, dress, eat, shit...I'll be that troll under the bridge; that chained, kidnapped kid in the basement closet. I am that faint voice heard trapped at the bottom of a sewer-pipe or mine shaft that nobody knows how to set it free.

Oh, there's Dad, the couch potato confined to his den. He doesn't see daylight that often. Immunocompromised in a Covid world, he rarely ventures through that portal to the real world.

How would I navigate the end of my and Dee's life on some new life stage? Maybe Dee figures out the rest on her own. All I can say is "sorry, we couldn't climax together."

31

A Game Changer?

Heeeeeey. Day 617 after first entering the hospital, we have a neurologist winning the diagnosis trifecta and willing to step up being comfortable rendering a specific diagnosis. In retrospect, it was more than an interesting and productive meeting with my NYU neurologist. Even though, as the doctor said, the known number of cases on record the world over, to date, with a combination of symptoms similar to mine can be counted on one hand, I was relieved that some "plan" of attack could be developed.

My debilitating illness has a name. And yes, it's Autoimmune, Autonomic Ganglionopathy (AAG), or to be more specific and confusing: Acute Idiopathic Dysautonomia and/or Autoimmune Autonomic Neuropathy—take your pick. I don't have a cold, a broken bone, or even the familiarity of cancer. When reviewing my case, even most professionals have that "SNL Californians moment" of aimlessly rolling their eyes to the sky.

The unique approach presented to date, which gives me some temporary optimism, is really about presenting a plan of attack. Although the doctor candidly admitted that he's basically a "duck out of water," along with all the rest of the other quackers, when it comes to dealing with my particular hybrid of neuropathy. He can address the discomfort related to my autonomic dysfunctions. He can simply re-prescribe medications in a fashion to alleviate the symptoms of bladder retention, blood pressure, sleep aid, weight gain, depression, and maybe even wishful-thinking sex issues. Along with the results of my sleep test, these things can provide some comfort of life even though the current science doesn't permit restoration pre-neuropathy. If you can't cure the illness, treat the symptoms. To that end, there is no nerve regeneration; no key of freedom from my jail-cell. No one to stop the rain. So, now I, along with the rest of the 70 million world-wide "junk drawer" sufferers, deal with that reality and the idea of at least being relatively comfortable, while there is no cure. But will the "new" quality of life be a fair enough trade-off for further suffering?

WHAT HAVE WE LEARNED FROM THIS ORDEAL?

To recap, it's been more than two years that I've been living with this Ganglionopathy, Dysautonomia, or whatever.

For one thing, I'm not alone in my handicapped condition. Although my illness was acute in nature, there are countless others with similar afflictions. However, after 70 years of a vibrant life, to have it suddenly transformed, is disconcerting at the least. You enter a hospital healthy but emerge a different entity. But how about for those around me? "With some of our misdirected and unreasonable, expectations today, I was tempted to say, "Alexa, make it all better." (You heard it here, first.)

I've learned that; particularly with an acute illness, the onset of the new environment can also induce the onset of panic. Waking up after the transformation, one asks: "How do I live like this?"

The murmured answer is to think of ending one's life because going forward in this diminished and transformed capacity is difficult and humiliating. But we all have as much right to be here as anyone else, I suppose. Get over it if you can. Finding love and support from the family, medical financial assistance to alleviate the stress of financial ruin and the unnecessary choice of what to pay for, are two immediate solutions alleviating unnecessary conflict. Seek out self-help groups familiar with PTSD and Facebook your particular health issue, even though they're no smarter than victims. Learn the tricks for the handicapped; the parking stickers and tags, the motorized carts, going to the head of the line, airport perks, and feistiness; which is without even mentioning the other options: learning to tie hangman's nooses; jerry rigging and disabling wheelchair brakes; even learning across-the-neck shaving with a barber's razor; oops! These are the guerrilla tactics that become necessary for patients with neuromuscular disorders to enable them to either stand up and be heard, or otherwise, take control of their destiny through their last option.

32

My Life, as I Knew it, is Over.

I realized my life, as I knew it, pre-June 2018, was over, never to return. So, in the last two years I've concluded that I can continue to drag around that corpse of dashed hopes, lamentations and anger of a life once lived and stolen, chasing a mythical cure, or I can be grateful for an extension of what I do have: the opportunity to live in my *afterlife*; the opportunity to resign myself to the futility of my condition going forward, and getting used to it under new and different circumstances. Another life, *after* my previous *life*.

People who live in the afterlife are those who have experienced a cataclysmic change. What is Death other than the irrevocable end to a life?

So, from that perspective, what is the difference between Death and a debilitating and transformative illness becoming permanent, yet we're compelled under duress to survive it? The *Afterlife* is what occurs after such a transformative event. Some may limit the afterlife to after death, or the fantasy of some resurrection (like Frankenstein), but they're ignoring the facts. When you're dead your corpus is disposed of after the goodbyes. Nothing further to talk about. You're simply someone's memory.

My afterlife is another life, a second life, an altered life, if you will, after my original life. My first born-life as lived and known until June 2018, was over. I had to commit suicide to not have to drag around that same corpse, post-morteming those dashed hopes, should'ves, would've, could'ves, anger and disappointment. I resigned myself to the unchangeable, and to my suicide when I concluded there was no place further to have optimism as to any sort of cure. The acceptance of my condition was the concession. At least there would be no groping-in-the-dark, blind hope anymore. No more self-inflicted misery searching for the unfindable. Move on.

The afterlife was a concept conceived by ancient inhabitants of the World to assuage those confronting brutal violence of combat that there would be a better place to greet and not fear what came next after death. So yes, I did commit suicide by accepting the end of my life as was lived. I moved on with whatever I still retained in my afterlife. I checked in through that place of the unknowable that separates one life from another.

Witness the deal with my death. I got a free ticket for that transitional period without the stress of bills, politics, and whatever else that may have previously bothered me. I have less "cares." No more artificial or arbitrary achievement standards. If I'm to be denied the option to live or not live under my own conditions, then I can choose what conditions I have to endure.

In my afterlife, I'm not compelled to really be a trailblazer when it comes to navigating the circumstances of my new life... Assuming I can endure the pain or discomfort, it then becomes learning about the ins and outs of maneuvering around my new obstacle path by inventing, sharing, or listening to those who precede me like everyone has since the dawn of time. Facebook Groups offer some clues and a place to commiserate, to not feel alone. But it helps to be taught the ropes. There should be classes, groups, meetings to "ease" or inform the new patient as to the incoming pitfalls; not to be cast to the wind to experience unaware what others have seen as steps and tripping points to come. It would certainly be productive for all to institute a short learning course for acute illnesses such as mine to be updated on expectations and strategies of what's to come. We stepped in shit—now what? Stay in a drifting rowboat or just pull the plug.

This has to come from something better than our current medical system. I've learned that the medical community is sometimes in over their heads as the science, or the medicine hasn't enabled them to catch-up with a disease. They can't even try to diagnose, let alone treat these illnesses. Despite their resources, they often fall far short of success. And they do overprescribe tests, medicines, and procedures in the interest of protecting their asses as a matter of overabundant caution. They just throw shit at the patient and see what sticks, or more or less stand idle, ultimately, waiting for a lightbulb to go on. Which, as to a cure, it doesn't.

Loved ones often have trouble with any concept of an afterlife for the afflicted. I've learned that Dee, for one, has a hard time discussing my discomfort with my current situation and or my being content to end my life. She shuts down the conversation by saying I always bring it up. But that becomes circular, because if she shuts down the conversation, we end up not resolving anything. This creates conflict for us in an otherwise harmonious environment. Does the discussion of the end of my life take away hope for her? Can't I get some help in seeing clearly through this ordeal? Ya just want some honesty as to the prospects—not a future of speculation, avoidance, and vapid hope like many find themselves, trapped. A discussion on: "what comes next?" and a humane plan of attack, would certainly be appropriate in a proactive way.

The afterlife can't be defined by the first life alone. I've learned that my purpose is not necessarily the store. Or scurrying around doing something else to keep busy. My real purpose is the guidance of my family and being the role model of a father confronting adversity.

In the Covid defined world, there is a desperate need for this role. In my tree-trunk of life there'll be an indelible mark in one of the rings indicating the influence of an outside event such as my virus.

But it is only one of many. There have been other shocks to the "system" that I've experienced. This one is just one of many that I have endured, and apparently survived. It won't be the last that humanity experiences.

The question is, will the world learn from it and how to prepare? It certainly won't be the same. Climate change is on the horizon, inequality, hunger, and poverty loom to sow more disruption. We can all deal with our local issues, but will we learn that everything isn't just about dollars and us. Now that the world is becoming "crammed" into the size of a "village," it's how we all learn to leverage our strengths to peacefully and prosperously progress and coexist.

The other day we celebrated my 71st birthday at home with the kids. Although under the Coronavirus umbrella, I also spent the day with numerous friends. Jesse had his friends text me best wishes, and Dee scheduled our friends to either call or video chat. One was even a drive-by with a "Happy Birthday" sign! That gave me an idea for a business. For a fee, of course, we can do drive-bys with a sign with any message, just like those planes at the summer shore with those trailing messages. In the meantime, during Covid limitations, we learn to abide and, helplessly, adjust to the new rules.

33

In my Head, not in a Bed.

Although typing is becoming more challenging, and injuries are mounting because the fainting is increasing, the energy is waning, and the hands are getting lost in the bedsheets. I am compelled to consider concluding this narrative. But some parting thoughts:

I've learned life's a highway with everyone zooming by on their motorcycles with a hail of bullets from beginning to end. Some get hit fatally and crash, others only get wounded along the way to the offramp. Others constantly enter and speed up. Apparently, along with my life's wounds, I along with my passengers, took a life-changing hit which compelled me to change lanes and slow down. A time to reflect on the distance and sights I've traveled before reaching my own exit.

I surrender. After 50+ years of newspaper delivery, snow shoveling neighbor's walks, cabana boy, parking lot attendant, the force majeure of Corona; I feel like throwing up my hands in resignation. I just don't have the mental strength. To me, shelter-in-place and the force majeure is about the final admission of defeat. I'm essentially grounded forever. Being immunocompromised, I'm not supposed to be exposed to foreign elements. That means possibly no vaccination and be in a bubble if going out.

I feel like I've been around long enough that the years and their significant events have passed me the same as sitting in H.G. Wells'

Time Machine. My eyes have seen the Vietnam War, multiple race riots, 19% prime lending and mortgage bank rates, dot.com bubbles, stock market crashes, real estate great recessions, moon walking, and now a pandemic. What's left remaining to experience that my pain can be ignored?

I remember the gas lines around the blocks because of the oil embargoes of the late 70's. Now, it's the lines to supermarkets and Covid testing sites, limiting the prescribed number of people because of social distancing, and hoarding. So, only a god knows what I'm going to miss. I'm tired. Do I have to live through the 10-minute war of 2027; the ensuing famine of 2031; the plague of 2035 or the painful death of a loved one? Extending life expectancy comes at a tremendous cost just because we can. And it can all be avoided in an instant. How much is enough to endure?

Although the Corona virus is a perfect cover for a couch potato with a compromised immune system, I'll do it on my own terms. I will proceed to my own drummer and pace. Home is everything. It's love, it's memories, it's safe. And as compromised as I am, why would I risk exposure and hang with the crowds of people of far less interest to me? The strength I have remaining isn't even worth the effort. "Been there..."

Looking back on my life, how did I get here? Surviving all the social and economic impacts with their game-changing scars. The three kids with their lacrosse, soccer and football, tennis lessons, summer camps and trips, bar mitzvahs, college plans; and all the bruises, broken teeth, and stitches in between.

I have no regrets. It's not about the pleasure of others. It's about what can you endure while giving a gift to others. Of course, as long as they aren't wishing you dead! It's one more time to guide the kids that, yes, "This too shall pass." And be a role model in the process.

With Corona, the kids visiting and staying over, have an opportunity to see how the parents are doing, but also to get their due kudos for current accomplishments. It's also a teaching moment for the parents and the kids to learn empathy and what may lay ahead for them and to also learn compassion for those in need.

I have a lot to show for what I have accomplished in life. My boys, my wife, my life, my happy homeowners, and Smoked customers. When we're open, it's always a family party. And now we're even getting repeat orders for our "hero" meals from our hospital first-liners and feed-the-needy from the Covid economic impact. Ya know, if they have a smile on their faces when returning to their shift, I'm happy to be a part of that.

34

Healthcare Rights in the Real World

According to the National Institutes of Health, animals also suffer from neuropathies and their related issues. But Mother Nature naturally addresses this issue. If I lived 10,000 years ago, I would have been culled from the herd and been somebody's dinner long ago.

We're facing a declining birthrate (not to mention a poor immigration policy curtailing the acquisition of needed help) ultimately resulting in a dwindling workforce. How about keeping our current workforce healthy? Won't that help our future problem? Infrastructure legislation requires millions of people to execute. If we have nothing but healthy, rich people, who's going to do the work? Who's going to build the infrastructure; or even be the babysitter? You want people to be self-sustaining? *Help* them to achieve that goal of self-sufficiency.

I'm all for profit. I loved making a profit when building houses or operating the restaurant. But there's a conflict when healthcare incentivizes profit. Aggressive doctors increase medical costs because they're in a for-profit mode. At the public's expense—they can't lose. But that's not sustainable.

It promotes aggressive treatment and duplication of testing and potential iatrogenic issues. A database with highlights of questionable actions can save millions from potential malpractice and unnecessary duplicate care. We certainly have the computing power. If you have the money one can, unquestionably, order the most expensive item on the menu. No one is taking our rights away on how to spend it. But if food and healthcare are basically utilities; they become human rights for which we all become responsible. The regulated Medicare system has difficulty competing within the free-for-all and sometimes chaotic for-profit system.

It's easy to pass the beggar and the homeless on the street because they're portrayed as "the others" with their own problems. But wouldn't it be better for all if we could figure out some system where all can survive and prosper? More buying power for the top 1% 's products.

It's outlandish! To believe some are more entitled than the rest is obsessively selfish. This illness, and others, were not our choices. So, why are we singled out to suffer when a possible cure or relief is sitting on some shelf and some people simply can't afford the expense? A byline in the *NYTimes*: "It's hard enough to have a child with cancer. It shouldn't crush families financially."

To make matters worse, except for paying some $20 copays to local doctors, after 3 months in the hospital, testing up the wazoo, IVIG for 6 months, plasma exchange, multiple MRI's and tests, etc., being on Medicare, I haven't looked at or paid anything else. HOW IS THAT POSSIBLE? It's noble to care for the elderly. But why only the less productive, and aged, get Medicare? What are we thinking?

Granted, I may be a guinea pig for all that are intrigued by my case, but what's the difference when it comes to suffering? Healthcare for some shouldn't be the roll of the dice or the luck of the draw when the 2020 Credit Suisse Global Wealth report reveals that the top one percent of households globally own 43 percent of all personal wealth, while the bottom 50 percent own only one percent. Change the paradigm from discriminating dogma, and return to the sustainable, nature's original system of: "evolved from creation;" as from that sulfur-based, single cell something or other formed more than 3 billion years ago from some "primordial soup."

There's something wrong with the system when doctors are taking marketing courses to increase their own sales and increase revenues. So, getting a second opinion only increases the likelihood of aggressive and excess tests of doctor's reviews thereby driving up the cost of the healthcare system. It's OK to get a second opinion. But it doesn't have to always start at square one with a new doctor duplicating new tests thereby adding additional costs which we all pay.

Maybe this pandemic is becoming a weeding out process for the nursing home shlunkers. But maybe they just don't have the strength to bother and if they could find the strength to raise their middle fingers to the world, maybe they would.

Maybe they would like to be "put to sleep" rather than confinement to satisfy the will of others. We do that for our pets! Why aren't nursing home folks, at least, afforded the option? Isn't it *their* lives they want to exercise some control over? Would those who want to end their lives be more enthusiastic about leaving some "buyout" money to the family as an inheritance instead of burning up Medicare payments while just keeping them alive? Pay them to leave the "party." I remember my mother almost sitting helplessly at the Nursing home consultation hardly having a say in her disposition. Not to mention being with some stranger with conflicting, profit-oriented interests?! Need the likes of a super-duper sound system; mud-flaps; undercoating; et al? Wouldn't many finding a few dollars be more appreciative of the funds than knowing the gov't delayed the inevitable by throwing money at an ungrateful almost-corpse? Time for a buyout to free up some space and resources.

Clean out the "deadwood." Ask Mom or Dad if they have a preference!

When Gma doesn't want to eat her bacon, it's time for a farewell cruise to the sun. If I could spare the bucks, I would commission a college grad to figure out the death insurance payout. Who wins, on multiple levels, is Medicare and the Government, insurance companies, and especially society. No round-trip ticket necessary. If Wall St. can analyze derivatives there's no reason that they wouldn't uncover a new business, one that can capitalize on giving "options" BACK to those who have been disadvantaged.

The system works against itself when it tries to salvage or extend the life of those who no longer want to live when expending untold sums to keep the near-vegetables alive. Where's the return on investment? We can't keep clogging up the end of the system with no relief. Don't force people to take an option they have no interest in by keeping them alive. Cultivating wheelchair Bingo teams is unsustainable. Stop clogging up the system at the end with the shlunkers waiting in their beds for their end!

Of course, nobody did an environmental impact statement before human-kind's brains and behavior were permitted to be included in the animal kingdom. Although a fascinating organ, some god didn't know the monster-brain they created. We've already screwed up the formula for peaceful harmony among neighbors and our environment. What's next—us? Instead of yearning for some "end of days" story to hasten our arrival at some fantasy playground for the dead, change the paradigm to making the world we live in a better place—today.

And if the misconceived dream IS to reach that playground with the likes of "dancing virgins"—why deny the choice? I'll take my chances. But I can hear the "wheelchair lobby" already when they realize sales are down because less are needed...

Think of it this way. We all perish from something. We don't live forever. We all have maladies from birth. Other problems sneak attacking us at any time later. Toward the end we're more prone to coming to a terminal phase. On the way, if we were observed in time lapse photography, we would see the slow decomposition of our bodies slowly disappearing and returning into the earth. "Ashes to ashes..."

We go through phases like all the other animals and living things on earth. No, we're not entitled to any different rewards than other living creatures, just because we're supposedly the most communicative. We're just expected to act our part in the ecological order. Our position on the food chain doesn't entitle us to bully its resources with wanton waste or abuse.

We all start aging from the beginning and go through phases of life until our natural lifespan comes to its end. We have been told stories created and motivated by our ignorance and fears of the unknown to assuage those fears. We're told, when we die, we go to a better place as a reward for good behavior or hell for inappropriate. So why do we delay the inevitable? Christianity has its Heaven or Hell, the Greeks and Romans' Elysian Fields, Ancient Egyptian's the Field of Reeds, not to mention, countless others with their own terminal "fantasy resorts." When in reality they were dealing with the disposal of biological matter also known as biological waste; what are the facts of life or are we fed beliefs for power and profit?

Why do we have the most primitive body disposal system? For possessing such intelligence it makes our name on a piece of paper and getting 200 SAT points look stupid. Where do all the dead animals go? They're recycled, cleaned off the earth, and room and resources made for the new. Instead, humanity developed a whole system of rituals contrary to nature's perfectly designed system. We're hoarders of the dead with a defective outmoded design for disposal. With the Human population expected to increase to 12 billion inhabitants, we'd better come up with a solution for more efficient processing of these transient lives. So why do we persist in pursuit of extending the near-dead lives when it's little more than shoveling shit against the tide? They're goners eventually.

Little more than saving the corpse. We don't throw old asphalt out from replacing our highway surfaces because it started taking up precious landfill space. So, we've learned to reuse the replaced material sometimes along with other recycled materials. Why are we fighting Mother Nature by trying to bulldoze all the mountains when we can build on top? Why do all departing souls get a piece of real estate to call their own? We'll look back one day and say, "what *were* we thinking?" As we continue to stockpile the billions of the dead in underground, covered, holes-in-the-ground, the cemetery landlords and box builders will have to adjust their business plans to accommodate a new way of thinking. Wow! What a radical and constructive way of operating.

A fundamental question arises from all the competition and polarization of our societies due to their own, anachronistic individually, perceived exceptionalism. But the time of that primitive mantra has passed. When maintaining laws and incentives on a nationalistic basis becomes counterproductive and interference to sustaining populations, it should be back to the drawing board—and decide how we *all* get along—as much hokum as that sounds to some. But war is not the answer to population control.

Why is the goal ultimately death or suffering to the loser when that cliché: "A rising tide raises all boats" has so much more appeal? This is the technological thinking age. Maintaining individual political and economic competing policies promoted by different societies becomes a waste of humankind's abilities. We shouldn't compete with chest-beating, tug-of-war-style, anymore for individual survival, but with solving problems that a growing and more intercon-nected earth's population now faces. Which is better? It's time to put all of those Master's Degrees to more practical use to solve our real problems.

You don't want to hear about my sexual preferences or fantasies? Why should I be more than amused about your religious fantasies and stories of dogmatic behaviors. Let's work collectively on solving problems that affect us all. Let's talk, candidly, about specifically, something that will affect every, man, woman, and child forever-more!

Most know that no one's getting out of life alive. But all of those connected to the system: doctors, pharmaceuticals, nursing facili-ties, etc. are competing for profits from defying that basic truth. They treat the nursing home shlunkers like sustainable cows. Make it worth their while to save on fruitless defiance of the obvious. Share the savings with a buyout for unnecessary future care. With a central database, a whole host of expense issues becomes more controllable while containing cost. Now, throw in a little AI (artificial intelli-gence) to solve some Iatrogenic issues, and now you're talking a sys-tem that makes some sense. Who knows; maybe even people will have a better chance of survival?

Take out the costly profit component and treat healthcare as a human right, or a utility; one that includes the right to die as well as live.

Not everyone needs 9 0's in their bank account. Most people want to know that they will be able to feed their families, can get ahead, and have a laugh or two or more on the way.

While authoring my previous book, *Our Road to Hatred, How we Raise our Bullies*, living in the U.S., and having traveled to third world countries, I realized that all people share human universals (common human traits). That along with some other science, confirms the equality of modern humanity regardless of appearance, place of origin, or whatever we've been lead to believe before. Part of revolutionizing this equation is a paradigm shift involving healthcare and basic human rights including education, opportunity, and security. And, if those who can game the system with tax breaks and other self-serving, perks; they can at least give the worker-bees healthcare, social security, a clean environment, and other safety nets. Then, the "gamers" can fuck with the system all they want; but, at least, there's downside protection for those who suffer from the "gamers" ill-fated decisions. Not, the luck of the partisan's choice. Currently, it seems like we're just a small step away from the futuristic *Hunger Games.*

Everyone doesn't aspire to have the riches of the Bill Gates', Warren Buffet's, or even the Donald Trumps. For many, just survival with those they care about would be satisfying enough.

35

If we're so smart, why are we cheugy?

If we have the wisdom and intelligence to create technology to communicate globally, then we can educate ourselves to self-sustainability, instead of practicing some 2,500-year-old ancient, rulebook of dogma to determine the course of our existence. Stop being so cheugy, you outdated hipsters! 2,500-year-old dogma is not trendy. It's old-fashioned, archaic thinking. First, we have to give up the imaginary deity-driven ideology that dictates and prevents us from, inclusively, solving this conundrum.

Free men don't have kings, so how can we stand to live at the discretion of a lord? If you're the servant of X, you're not free.

I see the likes of Gabby Gifford and see myself in her shoes. She has a voice, of some physical disability that was out of her control. If we have something to contribute, then find a way to make it heard. That's motivation enough to many. Those who can't endure the pain, it should be your choice; not laws guided by 2,500-year-old "sages."

From Maura Kelly's description in the *NY Times* "The Unknowability of Other People's Pain" is about the pain her father suffered leading to his suicide. It's about what chronic pain can lead to:

66 *"Mostly, though, the pain was so severe it kept me from* 99
thinking about anything else. Physical suffering will do
that. It "destroys a person's self and world," as Elaine
Scarry, a Harvard scholar, noted in her influential book
"The Body in Pain." It shrinks the universe and magnifies
the individual until the hurt becomes all there is."

In retrospect, to me, this has truly been a journey in courage. To those commiserating and in search of relief from your illnesses, you are the explorers in the unknown of where this leads us.

If you think of suicide, or now the more appropriate and PC, "physician-assisted dying," it's OK. If the pain outweighs the potential good, that's your assessment. It's your humanitarian right to determine your own fate. We're raised to fend for ourselves, make our own decisions, and "enjoy" the consequences. But we can't determine when we can stop being a pain-stricken, "rodent" on a legislated treadmill?

I have a pretty good idea of where this is going. My mother was 85 when she was bouncing off the walls in the middle of the night to pee. I'm 71 and now doing the same. I see the regression, as with my mother; from vibrancy, to cane, to walker, to wheelchair, to bedridden, to dead-in-the-bed.

If we are half genetic clones, to a degree, of our Parents, why then do we believe that we can't inherit some of our parental gene sequences. If my looks can be inherited, why can't some of the interior, illness-stuff also be? On the way the body starts to shut down. Acceleration of illness exceeds progress or maintenance of exercise or treatment. In other words, it's downhill from here. This ole' elephant is on its way to the boneyard. So, what's the point to tortuously prolong the costly, inevitable? I wouldn't interrupt nature's design for my cat or dog. It's expensive and futile.

The nursing home aisles are stuffed with wheelchair shlunkers. What is that common thread? "Oh, you can do it." Those famous words, like: "Nice try." to the kid swinging the bat at tee ball. I'm not seven or 27 in need of rehab. I'm 71 and prematurely shutting down as a recovery asset. I'm not trying to bench press 150 lbs. I can hardly do 5! You can tell a 10-year-old: "they can do it." Don't insult an adult; so, you can tolerate or visit them as infrequently as necessary to assuage your conscience? At least offer them to be cannabis stoned 24 hours a day. Let the family have a little joy for the misery on visiting day. What, Gma's going to be a heroin addict?! Picture it—a nursing home full of stoned, if not near-dead, shlunkers.

* * *

Why do we euthanize our pets? To put an injured or dying animal down is humane. Are we being humane with ourselves and other loved ones?

Why not be humane with humans? Was Dr. Frankenstein humane to Mr. F?

Will it come to a point when even others ask why am I being kept alive? For someone's entertainment or pleasure? Are we avoiding the prospect of the torment to come, or instead, of bond breaking, separation? The prospect of death torments the survivors more than the patients.

I remember my mother declining to go on the bar mitzvah Caribbean trip because she didn't have enough "spoons." Now, I get it. Simply, I think we're all just getting old. And aging is part of the dying process, our maladies with labels. Everyone suffers from something. We all have preexisting conditions at some time or other. Like the kids now "suffer" from the likes of ADHD or Bipolar; everyone requires a label to fit into some diseased or affected group. My kind falls into the junk draw of diagnosis's; Dysautonomia. But euphemistically more commonly known as a natural deterioration of bodily functions, aka aging and then dying. Heck, a 70 year-old person needs more maintenance than an automobile of the same age. We are all given an allotment of tableware when we enter the world. Who still has a complete set when our lives are over? This enormous grip around my body distracts from concentration and leads to exhaustion. How can I keep up the pace? Why am I compelled to try? That drawer of silverware, everyone starts out in life with, never looks the same at the end. Nature has its ways.

As Bertrand Russel argued, in his *The Will to Doubt;* you can't have progress if your thoughts and ideas are constrained by dogma. Open your mind to new ideas and imagine you were never taught about invisible deities and gods with their divisive, parochial, creeds. Instead, consider how we're all connected on this earth with a common goal of survival—but not when a winner takes all and stands alone. Imagine a lion could devour all living creatures without any natural, constricting controls. Humankind, alone, has that distinction. Unabated, someday maybe it will.

36

End game

I had another video meeting with the NYU crew. They finally were able to get in contact with Mayo and they agreed on the possible presence of another culprit. They believe that it could be the "T cells" that continue to go rogue. Like those Japanese soldiers from WWII still fighting a war on some of the forgotten islands who never got the message that the war was over. They'll prescribe and try an off-label drug used for Multiple Sclerosis. Imagine if in the future they can use something to tell the pawns, the T-cells, or the Japanese, for that matter, that the war is over, to redirect the autoimmune troops.

Having been on a high-school chess team, I see the next few moves in this game. I can be immunocompromised and be a bubble man. Now, I can go out and play in traffic on the freeway with the cars whizzing by; waiting to get hit in the age of Coronavirus. All legal. With the Coronavirus we've just reshuffled my deck of cards, options, and opportunities. What will I do?

Maybe we're looking at things the wrong way. Maybe Individual maladies we have, that become known as a disease, is really just the natural progression in the human condition of growing and then dying?

In the time lapsed photography of the visual of our lives, we see the picture morphing with time until death. Aging is the process of decomposition. Starting at birth, ripening, and becoming sweeter with age, but combined with our genetic links to predispositions, we all, randomly, return to the inherent natural elements around us.

The American Gothic couple, with the pitchfork, is an American picture of old age. The new sign is the picture of some old soul lying in a diaper, motionless in the bed, with one leg bent, and a peak at the bush with the blanket not completely covering the embarrassment. "Oh, this is my retirement and I'm just lounging?" When is enough, enough of this dehumanizing extension of life?

As for me, you can either cremate me which is not carbon and energy free or sustainable, or put me in a woodchipper and return me to the soil as fertilizer and say thanks to the other animals in the food system for allowing me to share their earth. Who knows, maybe the tomatoes will even taste better for the survivors? We are not supreme beings. We are just at the top of the system. We shouldn't exploit that position; but hold it responsibly.

We should give up whatever ideologies prevent us from solving this conundrum of unclogging the drain. Because, in the same way that denying birth control is not providing critical healthcare, preventing elective end-of-life ends up with a mess of an equation for a decent later life.

From: The NYTimes:

> "How long can we live?" "In any case, longevity scientists agree, significantly elongating life without sustaining well-being is pointless, and enhancing vitality in old age is valuable regardless of gains in maximum life."

"In her final years at La Maison du Lac, the once-athletic Jeanne Calment, [who lived to 122], was essentially immobile, confined to her bed and wheelchair. Her hearing continued to decline, she was virtually blind, and she had trouble speaking. At times, it was not clear that she was fully aware of her surroundings."

Where do we draw the line for "cruel and unusual punishment?" And to what end? Almost forget the patient; what about the survivors always living on that precipice of a loved-one's demise? When is the end to unrecoverable resources expended to stave off the inevitable? Maybe younger people full of vitality shouldn't be making laws about theirs, and others, future conditions of existence.

"Today, more people are surviving the major diseases of old age and entering a new phase of their life in which they become very weak," Robine said, "we still don't know how to avoid frailty."

Now, also, add to our conundrum, the unmentioned prospective cost of long-term care for those not living in nursing homes. How draining of funds and human resources just to keep the near-corpse alive at home? Are these the jobs we aspire to? Doesn't take much to realize that the health and pre-death jobs associated with humanity's current formula for end-of-life care is unsustainable; not to mention just plain senseless. Just keep combing Mom's hair and wiping Dad's chin—while making sure the diapers are changed, forever? Is that my future—yours perhaps?

Doesn't it come down to "herd" management and the necessity to normalize the situation? If we are going to present ourselves as supreme creatures, then we are to responsibly (sustainably) steward and manage our ecosystem. Meanwhile, the shlunkers play along with the "gotta keep 'em breathing charade" until responsible people ease the shlunkers out of their misery. Nothing works well when it's constipated. Don't block the system.

So, this was my solution. My life as I had known until the age of 69 was over. I committed suicide and moved on in my afterlife. Just a warmup to the final act. There're no dancing virgins after death. If you're lucky maybe in the afterlife with a "rub 'n a tug"—but not in the time after death. So, hurry, hurry if one is so inclined.

I miss the spontaneity and intimacy of a sex life. Now all that remains alive are the memories. My thoughts now become more directed at problem solving. Does it become a choice to sit down and discuss, as mature individuals, that I resign myself to hanging up the baseball mitt and cleats, or consider outsourcing something as innocent as a medicinal hand job? Maybe I can simply still try to throw the ball. And if I can, why not? I can still search for *my* holy grail.

Forget the taboo and deterrent of a religious overlay. It's not about having sex or loving another. The therapist is no different than the pastry chef or the manicurist. The same as the pet, dog, going to the vet to have "the glands" cleaned. And just because two individuals needs aren't in sync possibly because of age and circumstances, doesn't mean we hang up the cleats altogether. But many of the disabled can still have the desire and need for a good organism leading to self-worth and better mental health. Less depression?

Either give the disabled the tools to value their existence, or the right to terminate their misery of a chronically painful and unvalued life. Netherlands, Sweden, and Germany, among others, offer assistance following the guidelines of The United Nations Convention on the Rights of Persons with Disabilities and its Optional Protocol. Other countries take up the conversation.

From: The United Nations Department of Economic and Social Affairs Disability:

> "The Convention follows decades of work by the United Nations to change attitudes and approaches to persons with disabilities. It takes to a new height the movement from viewing persons with disabilities as "objects" of charity, medical treatment and social protection towards viewing persons with disabilities as "subjects" with rights, who are capable of claiming those rights and making decisions for their lives based on their free and informed consent as well as being active members of society."

If we can't provide a life with choices to minimize the cost and the prolonged misery, then why is it acceptable to, in essence, do nothing but watch an "old dog" take its last breaths?

Dysautonomia, which is the dysfunction of the Autonomic Autoimmune Nervous system (AAN), or neuropathy affecting those components, is the next cancer. It's also known as the "Invisible disease," because from the outside, all looks well. It's the umbrella like heart disease encompasses many unnoticeable subcomponents of failure—high blood pressure; low; hardening of the arteries; I don't know them all. But it is now coming closer to understanding the micro components of what happens when we reach the ends of our life expectancy; Neuropathy apparently, being a significant culprit. Dysfunction, or dysautonomia of our life sustaining systems appears to be a natural progression toward the end of our lives. And with the diagnoses of Dysautonomia, comes another label: "disabled."

Hamlet's question: "to be or not to be" refers to his not staying alive and his fear of what would his existence be with overthinking the alternative—his unknown world of death. He is considering death to avoid facing something he is afraid of. My dilemma doesn't fear the alternative, the world of "that undiscovered country," but demands the guiltless, acceptance, as well as the right to proactively cross that threshold of one's painful existence to end it. I fear my jail cell to-come before I'm fed to the tomatoes.

In some strange way, I'm ok having the end of my life being defined in a secure, controlled, way. I only advocate for a choice and regulated method of assisted-termination, while avoiding the unregulated violence—a method to end whose lives suffer beyond that threshold of the acceptable.

I don't want to have disagreements with the kids, the wife; I've had enough. With this illness I can feel marginalized because I'm compromised in my ability to have a conversation or a previous "normal" life. If one doesn't have fluidity of thought because the diminution of executive function hinders same, why am I still on the playing field? Instead, I'm relegated to some wheelchair shlunker's queue.

Self-elected "Death with Dignity" would be doing you all a favor rather than having to live with the conflict of accepting my trauma producing, clandestine, and maybe messy, abrupt end. How dare anyone sentence me to a prolonged, tortuous death. Only I can stop this misery. But why do I have to do it unsupervised and alone? Until then, living in my afterlife gets me through the day.

Next stop on that train to death-land, is peace in itself, with the inevitable yet to come knowing I didn't miss anything.

It's not about longevity for the sake of a Guinness' world's record. It's about quality of life. *That* should be a personal choice.

* * *

So, after I recently ate a chunk of chocolate, pot-edibles, Dee and I had like a first date in two years, but this time without the Groucho mustache-glasses disguise. My needle moved. Miracles anybody? A spark? It was reminiscent of reading and completing my first elementary school book for which I felt so proud after completing— "The Chocolate Touch." But don't get too ahead of ourselves, it was all about the connection of the touch, this time, not the book. Now, in uncharted territory, while a poon-dog at heart... and with always the right woman, I may have to reconsider my current plans...

So, with the excited anticipation of searching for my hermit crab, some 35 years later, and, with **the** only love in my afterlife, giddily, like a dog on a leash with a mission, and an edible or two, Vavavavoom we go!

37

Epilogue

That ending is my fantasy—*my* 72 dancing virgins (or raisins). And I bought in. After 35 years, I remain insanely attracted to the crush of my life, my wife. All the maternal instincts a patient could want. She's sexy, giggly and fun. All that a guy could dream.

But regardless of however this ends, the end won't be about how courageous I was and I "lost my battle with..." because everyone "loses" their battle. But the end is not going to be about the last unwritten chapter of my life. Either the one with all the mess created by a failing body or one executed. I do know, if that's my intended fate, I'll figure out how to stop my sun from rising. This is *my* life:

> What right does anyone have to determine
>
> how I live
>
> The End
>
> of my life?

So, Dee took me for my first pedicure and foot massage. Isabella said, "Come back in a month." We're working on the other massage.

ACKNOWLEDGEMENTS

Thank you to my family for making the best attempt at empathizing with the invisible crank that I am...and

Thank you to Stephen Axtell at Kismet Writing and Development who assisted in the editing process; giving my story some coherence; and Nicole and Julie-Ann at the Pickawoowoo Publishing Group who helped make the publishing process so much easier.

CPSIA information can be obtained
at www.ICGtesting.com
Printed in the USA
BVHW060829291221
625055BV00016B/1317